INSULIN RESISTANT DIET

2 Manuscripts: Insulin Resistance Diet, Insulin Resistance Cookbook, Bonus - Plant Based Diet Cookbook

KATYA JOHANSSON

COPYRIGHT © 2016
ALL RIGHTS RESERVED

TABLE OF CONTENTS

INSULIN RESISTANCE DIET:

Introduction 2
Advantages of Insulin Resistance Recipes 5
1. Healthy Salmon and Mussels in Foil Parcel 8
2. Delicious Chicken Casserole... 9
3. Amazing Meal..10
4. Amazing Soy Zucchini Noodles 12
5. Healthy Garlic Parmesan Chicken and Zucchini............ 13
6. Amazing Eggplant, Squash & Zucchini Casserole 14
7. Delicious Salsa Chicken.. 16
8. Delicious Mediterranean Chicken................................ 17
9. Amazing Sticky Chicken 18
10. High Fiber Bread 20
11. Smoked Turkey Salad with Soy-lime Dressing..............22
12. Noodle Soup with asparagus, chicken stock, turkey.... 24
13. Healthy Bean with Tofu, Peanut, and Broccoli............ 26
14. Healthy Green Beans and Dumpling Soup 28
15. Healthy Salmon Burger 29
15. Healthy Vegetables with 3-Bean Salad 30
16. Amazing Lettuce Wrap Chicken.................................32
17. Healthy Pumpkin Soup 34
18. Amazing Granola Muesli 37
19. Healthy Banana Breakfast Drink 38
20. Delicious Fried Chicken 39
21. Amazing Moussaka 40
22. Tasty Lentil Sauce 42
23. Healthy Potato and Carrot Bake 44
24. Healthy Apple and Raisin Cake 46
25. Tasty Sweet Potato and Date Cake 48
26. Pasta with Lentil Marinara Sauce.............................. 50
27. Healthy Cherry Tomato and Brown Rice Salad with Artichoke Hearts 51
28. Berry Mousse 52
29. Blood Sugar Balancer...53
30. Healthy Meal...54
30. Tasty Chipotle Cashew Topping.................................56
31. Tasty Creamy Chipotle Chia 57
32. Tasty Smoked Salmon Wraps 58

33. Amazing Sweet Potato Muffins 59
34. Amazing Crumpets 61
35. Healthy Berry Yogurt Mousse 62
36. Creamy Tomato Soup 63
37. Tasty Tomato Sauce 65
38. Tasty Grill Sauce 67
39. Tasty Curried carrot soup 69
40. Amazing Red Tomato Salsa 71
41. Green Smoothie 72
42. Tasty Chicken, Mushroom and Porcini Soup Recipe ... 73
43. Healthy Broccoli and Turmeric Soup 74
44. Tasty Chicken and Vegetable Zoodle Soup 75
45. Tasty Sushi Roll Recipe 76
46. Healthy Wholesome Vegetable Stock 77
47. Tasty Turmeric Tea Golden Milk Recipe 78
48. Tasty Burrata with Rocket and Cherry Tomatoes 79
49. Tasty Basturma Egg Cups 80
50. Tasty Zucchini and Squash Bake 81

PLANT BASED DIET COOKBOOK:

Introduction 83
BREAKFAST RECIPES 85
1. Healthy Pumpkin Pancakes 85
2. Healthy Groovy Green Smoothie 87
3. Amazing Tofu Scramble 88
4. Amazing Potato Pancakes 89
5. Delicious Soy Yogurt 90
6. Amazing Power Porridge 91
7. Low Fat Tasty Cinnamon Nut Granola 92
8. Healthy Oat and Quinoa Cereal 94
9. Sweet Healthy Potato Hash Browns 95
10. Healthy Pumpkin Chia Pudding 96
11. Amazing Muesli 98
12. Chocolate Chip Tasty Pumpkin Muffins 99
DRESSING RECIPES 101
13. Healthy Vegan Mushroom Gravy 101
14. Delicious Tahini Dressing 103
15. Healthy Green Goddess Dressing 104
16. Healthy Mexican Salad with Lime Cilantro Dressing . 105
DESSERT RECIPES 107
17. Tasty Baked Pears with Cardamom 107
18. Amazing Raspberry Jello 108
19. Healthy Strawberry Ice Cream 109

20. Chocolate Chip Tasty Chickpea Cookies 110
21. Indian Spicy Carrot Pudding..111
22. Blueberry Lemon Tasty Coconut Bars 113
23. Health Black Bean Brownies 115
LUNCH RECIPES 116
24. Gluten-Free Tasty Sandwich Bread 116
25. Roasted Tasty Buddha Bowl 118
26. Tasty Vegetable Fritters 120
27. Healthy Bean and Vegetable Chili.............................. 121
28. Tasty Jackfruit Chicken Noodle Soup 122
29. Bean Sald 124
30. Tasty Tabbouleh 125
31. Delicious Red Pepper, Chickpea and Spinach Soup ...126
32. Spicy Tasty Hummus 128
33. Healthy Chickpea, Lentil and Spinach Stew..............129
34. Amazing Spicy Bean Spread 131
DINNER RECIPES... 132
35. Healthy Crispy Cauliflower... 132
36. Healthy Potato Lentil Turmeric Soup 134
37. Five Minute Fresh Tasty Salsa 136
38. Tasty Baked Sesame Fries 137
39. Healthy Chickpeas and Rice 138
40. Tasty Peanut Butter from Scratch 139
41. Amazing Creamy Mushroom Pasta 141
42. Delicious Vegan Pizza... 143
43. Tasty Alfredo Potato Bake 145
44. Healthy Black Bean with Potato Seitan Roast............ 147
45. Vegan Cheesy Sweet Potato & Kale Bake....................149
46. Healthy Chickpea with Potato Burger Patties.............151
47. Amazing Pea and Mushroom Risotto........................ 153
48. Amazing Seitan Roast 155
49. Roasted Garden Vegetables.. 156
50. Curried Delicious Rice Noodles................................. 157

INSULIN RESISTANCE COOKBOOK:

INTRODUCTION.. 161
Breakfast recipes 163
Lunch recipes 175
Dinner Recipes 189
Desserts 205
CONCLUSION 220

INSULIN RESISTANCE DIET

50 Delicious Recipes That Can Aid In Weight Loss, Reduce Insulin Resistance And Help Prevent Prediabetes

BY

Katya Johansson

More Books At:
www.katyajohansson.com

Copyright © 2016 by Katya Johansson.
All Rights Reserved.

INTRODUCTION

Insulin resistance as its name recommends is a condition where the body's reactions to the impacts of insulin are diminished. The body begins opposing insulin and along these lines the hormone insulin whose essential part is to bring down the glucose level can't work successfully. Insulin Is critical for the body's digestion system, all the more so the digestion system of proteins, fats and starches. It additionally assumes a key part in cell development and direction in the body. At the point when the body experiences this condition, it requires an expanded measure of insulin in light of the fact that the ordinary level insulin is not adequate for typical working.

The body opposes its own insulin and in addition remotely directed insulin. Weariness, laziness, hypertension, weight pick up, melancholy, hypoglycemia and fart are side effects to pay special mind to. Despite the fact that these indications are not restrictive to persons experiencing insulin resistance, they ought to be accounted for to the specialist quickly.

An insulin resistance eating routine is encouraged to people with this condition. This eating routine is like the eating regimen suggested for diabetic. The fundamental point is to standardize the glucose level. The starch and sugar admission is constrained. Proteins and great fats are added to the insulin resistance diet. Complex carbs and sugars are informed rather regarding straightforward ones, since they are assimilated rapidly into the circulatory system. It is imperative to constrain the fast ascent in the blood glucose level. Insulin resistance diet arrangement will incorporate 40-60% of starches, 20-30% of proteins and 20-30% of fat.
An insulin resistance diet menu ought to be without refined sugars and starches, boring carbs.

INSULIN RESISTANCE

The insulin resistance nourishment arrangement ought to be such that it helps switching insulin resistance. It should likewise keep away from the quick increment in the blood glucose level with a specific end goal to keep up a low level of insulin. The principle Insulin resistance diet nourishments are natural products, steamed and crude vegetables, for example, cabbage, tomato, celery, cucumber, cauliflower, broccoli and avocado, vegetables, for example, soya bean, beans and peas, fish and poultry and oils with crucial unsaturated fats, for example, olive oil, canola oil and flaxseed oil. Insulin resistance nourishments to maintain a strategic distance from are potatoes, pumpkins, bread, pasta, corn, red meat, organic products with a high sugar content and seared sustenance. These nourishments decline the condition by creating a quick ascent in the insulin level in the body. Insulin resistance diet nourishments should likewise be rich in fiber. In this manner around 25 grams of fiber must be devoured once a day. Apples, Pears, lentils and almonds are rich wellsprings of fiber. It is anything but difficult to discover insulin resistance nourishment records which give a smart thought about the quantity of calories, the glycemic file, and so forth that every sustenance contains.

Insulin resistance diet formulas can be made fascinating by taking after the trade framework. In this framework there is no meticulous calorie numbering. In this framework comparable nourishments fall under one class and sustenances in one gathering will have increasingly or the less the same amount if fat, protein, sugars and a comparative calorie content. Thusly one serving of a specific nourishment can be exchanged for a serving of another "comparative" sustenance. Nonetheless, it is essential to stick to the insulin resistance diet sustenance list when taking after such trade frameworks.

It is regularly watched that insulin resistance nourishments that assistance turning around the state of insulin resistance are likewise gainful for individuals with weight issues. Frequently large amounts of insulin build the fat generation in the body. To

KATYA JOHANSSON

add to the issue, insulin resistance and sustenance desires are additionally specifically related. Since this condition causes irregularity in blood glucose levels, the cerebrum gets signals that the living being requires nourishment regardless of the fact that it is not the situation. Henceforth the insulin resistance eating regimen and weight reduction go as an inseparable unit. Sound dietary propensities consolidated with consistent activity are valuable in battling the issue of IR and corpulence.

INSULIN RESISTANCE

ADVANTAGES OF INSULIN RESISTANCE RECIPES

The Insulin Resistance Diet that was endorsed to me permits the accompanying:
Vegetables – Eat Your Greens, Well Not All Greens...
You can browse the accompanying: broccoli, zucchini, eggplant, carrots, capsicum, celery, cucumber, lettuce, tomato, onion, shallot, leeks, green beans, asparagus, bok choy, choy entirety, snow peas, mushrooms, bean grows, horse feed grows, rhubarb, leeks, chives and on the off chance that you can stomach them, you can have cauliflower, Brussel sprouts and cabbage.

At first it appears to be restricting however there's sufficient assortment here to make a dinner delicious and not simply satisfactory.

Sauces, Condiments and Hello Flavor

Most general store purchased sauces and toppings have sugar included or utilized as an additive so I have taken to checking the name when I'm shopping.
The rundown incorporates soy sauce, fish sauce, clam sauce (I'm as of now considering Asian style dishes), tomato glue, a whiff of vinegar, lemon/lime juice, mustard and Worcestershire sauce.

The Spices of Life

I was calmed to discover that a large portion of the herbs and flavors I utilize are permitted, for example, garlic, thyme, oregano, bunch garni, basil, rosemary, ginger, bean stew, turmeric, nutmeg, pepper and paprika.
Soups

KATYA JOHANSSON

The rundown I was given peruses like a doctor's facility menu sheet so I will save you that. You can have clear soups, miso soup, stock 3D shapes and vegetable soup produced using the permitted list above.

Non-Alcoholic Drinks

We know we should drink no less than 2 liters a day yet I think that its hard to guzzle even 50% of that in summer. Tea, espresso, herb tea and water will turn into your closest companions. A little tomato juice is permitted, around 1/4 of a glass however ensure you purchase a brand that has no additional sugar.

Dessert/Fruit

Surprisingly in my life, I was advised not to eat natural product. It's all concentrated sugar. For the most part, a constrained determination of berries is permitted like strawberries, blackberries, blueberries, raspberries and the odd passionfruit. On the off chance that you're pondering what you can eat for treat, the answer is... nothing.
Shouldn't something be said about Artificial Sweeteners and Diet Products?
The eating regimen takes into consideration manufactured sweeteners, and items made with them, for example, diet jam, diet heartfelt, count calories soda (truly?) et cetera. My inclination is to abandon the counterfeit flavor and compound components that give the figment of sweetness with a sharp persistent flavor.

Hold tight... shouldn't something be said about Dairy?

Journal has been my issue with this eating regimen. I don't drink milk and I don't care for yogurt or the common Greek style yoghurts much. My calcium consumption has dependably

INSULIN RESISTANCE

originated from eating cheddar. Brie, Blue Cheese and Vintage Cheddar are among my top choices. However, cheddar has a high fat (and cholesterol substance to those tallying) and I was prompted not to eat it.

Osteoporosis keeps running in my family so I was not set up to surrender cheddar inside and out while on this eating routine. In the wake of begging my pro, I was permitted to eat 25g of cheddar a day as an evening nibble. You'll be reacquainted with your disregarded kitchen scales.

Different Exclusions – Wait... there's additional?

We realize that we are to lessen/cut down on carbs altogether from our eating regimen. That implies no white bread, pasta, rice, noodles, potatoes, pumpkin and sweet potatoes, kumera, and turnips, and the sweet fulfillment that originates from such delights. Be that as it may, did you realize that corn, peas and beetroot are likewise out?

Include a bean blend, cannellini beans, red kidney beans, chickpeas, hommus, quinoa, and lentils (an exceptionally constrained amount of lentils on the odd event) to the limited rundown, and take a full breath.

It's not the apocalypse but rather I took a gander at it as an opportunity to experience the storeroom and the refrigerator and

1. Healthy Salmon and Mussels in Foil Parcel

Ingredients

- 2 x 150g salmon filet
- 2 teaspoons of olive oil
- salt and pepper
- 1 zucchini, cut thin the long way
- 4 vast leaves of bok choy
- 4 dark mussels
- 2 cherry tomatoes, divided

Method

1. Preheat broiler to 160C.
2. On a vast bit of foil, layer the Ingredients in the accompanying request: zucchini, bok choy, salmon filet, salt and pepper, bok choy once more, dark mussels, cherry tomatoes.
3. Bring the edges of the foil together to shape a shut bundle.
4. Heat in the stove for 15 mins.

2. Delicious Chicken Casserole

Ingredients

- 300g incline chicken bosom, cut into lumps
- 2 tablespoons olive oil
- 2 cloves garlic, minced
- 2 cloves garlic, peeled and entirety
- 2 vast zucchinis, split lengthways and cut into pieces
- 6 mushrooms, quartered
- 6 set dark olives
- 1 small, onion cleaved
- ½ glass chicken stock
- 1 glass tomato sauce
- 2 sprigs crisp thyme
- 1 sprig tarragon
- 1 sprig rosemary
- bunch basil clears out
- slashed parsley for trimming

Method

1. In a broiler evidence goulash dish, chestnut the chicken in olive oil then set aside.
2. In the same goulash dish, delicately sauté the onion, zucchini, mushrooms and minced garlic in olive oil.
3. Include the tomato sauce, chicken stock and herbs.
4. Cover and cook in 160C broiler for 30 minutes.
5. Evacuate cover and cook for an additional 10 minutes.
6. To serve, sprinkle with slashed parsley.

3. Amazing Meal

INGREDIENTS

- ½ carrot, cut into meager strips
- ½ zucchini, cut into meager strips
- 2 mushrooms, meagerly cut
- bunch of infant spinach
- 2 shallots, cut into meager strips
- 2 segments of dried ocean growth, cut into slim strips
- ¼ cup cauliflower rice

TO COOK VEGETABLES:
- Sesame oil
- Soy sauce
- Toasted sesame seeds

BULGOGI MARINADE:
- 2 tablespoon soy sauce
- 1 tablespoon sesame oil
- 1 tablespoon Korean stew glue
- 200 g meat, daintily cut
- 1 egg yolk

METHOD

1. Cut meat into dainty strips and marinade in Bulgogi sauce.
2. Set all up vegetables.
3. Cook rice and keep warm.
4. Get ready cauliflower rice.

INSULIN RESISTANCE

5. Heat. Little sesame oil in dish, include every vegetable with a dash of soy sauce and cook on tender warmth for 2-3 minutes.
6. Put aside independently and keep warm.
7. Heat somewhat vegetable oil in a skillet and panfry the meat then keep warm.
8. Include. Little sesame oil to the same cup and cook rice for 2-3 minutes.
9. Amass dish: include a little sesame oil base. Top with rice. Include cooked vegetables and meat like spokes of a bike wheel. Sprinkle with sesame seeds.
10. Deliberately include the egg yolk in the center.
11. Present with a side of hot sauce.
12. To serve, combine all.

4. Amazing Soy Zucchini Noodles

Ingredients

- 2 zucchinis, spiralised
- ½ teaspoon oil
- Sauce:
- ¼ cup soy sauce
- 1 tablespoon of rice vinegar
- 1 tablespoon sesame oil
- ½ teaspoon crisply ground ginger
- toasted sesame seeds

Method

1. For the sauce, consolidate soy sauce, rice vinegar, sesame oil and ground ginger in a dish and blend well.
2. Heat ½ teaspoon of oil in a cup and delicately saute the zucchini noodles for 2 minutes.
3. Expel from warmth and add enough of the sauce to coat.
4. Serve as a side dish.

5. Healthy Garlic Parmesan Chicken and Zucchini

Ingredients

3 medium zucchini, cut
12 ounces chicken bosom or tenderloin, slashed
1 tablespoon garlic, finely slashed
1 tablespoon onion, slashed
2 glasses cut mushrooms
1/3 glass ground parmesan cheddar

Method

Shower a skillet or griddle with cooking spray and swing to medium/high warmth. Include onions and garlic, saute until they start to turn brilliant cocoa. Include the mushrooms and zucchini. Saute until mushrooms and zucchini begin to wind up delicate. Add chicken and keep on sauting on high warmth until chicken is totally cooked. Include the parmesan cheddar, mixing much of the time and covering every one of the pieces. Expel from warmth once cheddar has covered all pieces and dissolved to your preferring.

KATYA JOHANSSON

6. Amazing Eggplant, Squash & Zucchini Casserole

Ingredients

- 1.5 Yellow Squash, cut into 1/2" cuts
- 1 Medium Zucchini, cut into 1/2" cuts
- .5 Medium Eggplant, cut into 1" 3D squares
- .5 Medium Yellow Onion, sliced
- 2 cloves of Garlic, minced
- 1 10oz cup of Rotel (or whatever other diced tomatoes with chilies)
- .5 cup Canned Diced Tomatoes
- .5 cup ground Parmesan cheddar
- .5 cup shredded 2% Mexican Blend cheddar
- Spread Flavored Non-Fat Cooking Spray
- Garlic Salt
- Pepper

Method

1. I cooked this in a toaster stove. Preheat broiler to 400. Line a preparing dish with foil and spray with cooking shower to avoid staying (and SUPER simple tidy up!).
2. Warm expansive nonstick skillet over medium warmth. At the point when skillet is hot, coat with cooking spray. Include onions and garlic. Sautee until delicate. Include Rotel, diced tomatoes, eggplant, squash, and zucchini to skillet. Sprinkle with garlic salt and pepper to taste. Sautee for 5 minutes.

INSULIN RESISTANCE

3. Layer the eggplant/squash blend and Parmesan, rotating until eggplant blend is no more. Top with outstanding Parmesan (assuming any) and the Mexican mix cheddar. Prepare for 20 minutes (or until veggies are cooked to wanted doneness).

7. Delicious Salsa Chicken

Ingredients

- 5 Chicken bosoms
- 1 16 oz. cup La Victoria Thick'N Chunky mellow salsa
- 1/2 bundle Lawry's Taco Seasoning

Method

1. Trim fat from chicken. Wash chicken and spot chicken in Crock pot.
2. Sprinkle 1/2 bundle of taco flavoring onto chicken
3. Pour salsa over chicken.
4. Cook on low in simmering pot 6 to 8 hours.

8. Delicious Mediterranean Chicken

Ingredients

- 2 mugs slashed portabello mushroom (6 oz)
- 6 roma tomatoes, cleaved
- 1-14 oz can Reese Artichoke Hearts (6-8 medium estimated) quartered - depleted and flushed
- 1-4.25 oz can Mario Black Olives, slashed
- 1 Tbsp slashed garlic
- 2 Tbsp corn starch
- 1 lb. skinless/boneless (75 mg sodium/serving) chicken bosom - cut into pieces
- 1 Tbsp. dried italian flavoring (HERBS, not a "flavoring parcel")
- 1 glass College Inn (half less sodium) Chicken Broth Light and Fat Free

Method

1. Spritz slower cooker/simmering pot with Olive Oil non-stick shower.. Consolidate mushrooms, tomatoes, artichoke hearts, garlic and olives. Combine tenderly. Sprinkle with corn starch. Place chicken on top, sprinkle with Italian Seasoning. Include stock.
2. Cover and cook on low for 6 - 8 hours, on high for 3-1/2 to 4 hours. (Blend about part of the way through)
3. Present with entire wheat pasta (I utilized egg noodles)

9. Amazing Sticky Chicken

INGREDIENTS

- 1 teaspoon salt
- 2 teaspoons paprika
- 1 teaspoon cayenne pepper
- 1 teaspoon onion powder
- 1 teaspoon thyme
- 1 teaspoon white pepper
- 1/2 teaspoon garlic powder
- 1/2 teaspoon dark pepper
- 1 expansive cooking chicken (3-4 lbs.)
- 1 glass cleaved onion

METHOD

1. In a little bowl, completely join every one of the flavors. Expel giblets from chicken, clean the depression well and pat dry with paper towels. Rub the zest blend into the chicken, both all around, ensuring it is equally conveyed and down profound into the skin. Place in a resealable plastic sack, seal and refrigerate overnight.
2. At the point when prepared to meal chicken, stuff depression with onions, and spot in a shallow heating dish. Cook, revealed, at 250° F for 5 hours. After the primary hour, season the chicken once in a while (each half hour or thereabouts) with skillet juices. The cup juice will begin to caramelize on the base of the dish and the chicken will turn brilliant chestnut. On the off chance that the chicken contains a pop-up thermometer,

INSULIN RESISTANCE

disregard it. Let chicken rest around 10 minutes before cutting.

10. HIGH FIBER BREAD

INGREDIENTS

- 2 cups rye flour
- 2 Tbsp wheat gluten
- 1/2 cup oat wheat
- 1/4 cup moved oats
- 1/4 cup flax feast, more wheat, or 9-grain oat
- 1 Tbsp nectar
- 1 Tbsp olive oil
- 1 tsp salt
- 1 tsp bread yeast
- 1 tsp caraway or nigella seeds for included flavor
- 1 and 1/4 cup tepid water

METHOD

1. By including the gluten, you can escape with utilizing a much higher rate of entire grain and fiber while as yet getting batter that ascents in a bread machine. I have found that by taking after an essential proportion of 2 glasses entire flour (wheat, rye, oat, and so forth.) to 1 cup coarser Ingredients (wheat, oat, or rice grain, 9 grain oat, moved oats, seeds, and so on) alongside that additional gluten, the bread more often than not turns out firm and thick, yet not heavy or excessively dry. You may need to change the measure of water by a tablespoon or two relying upon your decision of grains. The nectar helps the yeast rise, so including more makes a more permeable bread. The oil keeps the bread from drying out subsequent to preparing, so the roll holds a new composition for a few days in the wake of heating.

INSULIN RESISTANCE

2. On the off chance that preparing this by hand, ply for around 10 minutes, let ascend for two hours, tenderly punch down, let rise again for 60 minutes, and heat for 60 minutes at 350 F.

KATYA JOHANSSON

11. Smoked Turkey Salad with Soy-Lime Dressing

Ingredients

- 1/2 glass shredded smoked turkey (~50 grams)
- 6 lances asparagus
- 1/2 glass purple post beans or green beans. (8 or so cases)
- 3-4 vast external leaves of margarine lettuce
- 1/8 cup pulverized toasted almonds.
- 1 tsp sesame seeds
- 1/4 cup coarsley cleaved cilantro

Dressing:
- 2 Tbsp nectar
- 1 Tbsp soy sauce
- 1 Tbsp Tiparos fish sauce (discretionary)
- 1 Tbsp Mirin rice wine
- 1 Tbsp sesame oil
- 3 new limes – squeezed (around 1/2 cup juice)

Method

1. For the dressing, in a fired or glass dish, warm the nectar in a microwave with the soy, fish sauce and rice wine for around 30 seconds. Mix to disintegrate the nectar. Include lime juice, and afterward wisk in the sesame oil just before serving.
2. For the vegetables, cut asparagus lances down the middle if fundamental, expel strings from the edges of

INSULIN RESISTANCE

the post bean cases and place all of them in a microwave safe dish that has a tight cover. Sprinkle a couple of tablespoons of the dressing over the vegetables, cover and steam in microwave for around 4 minutes, or until daintily cooked (still a bit crunchy).

3. Meanwhile, wash and sufficiently dry substantial external leaves of spread lettuce to stack around 3 or 4 on every plate, making a wide palatable dish. Sprinkle generously with cilantro. Stack a hill of smoked turkey in the middle. Organize the warm vegetables on the sides, shower with the fluid from the vegetable steaming dish, top with squashed almonds and dust with sesame seeds. Add extra soy-lime dressing if coveted.

12. NOODLE SOUP WITH ASPARAGUS, CHICKEN STOCK, TURKEY

INGREDIENTS

- 2 Carbs
- 3 Protein
- 1/2 cup cooked soba noodles (Japanese buckwheat noodles)
- 2 cups chicken soup
- 1 Tbsp soy sauce
- 2 Tbsp Tiparos fish sauce
- 1 Tbsp Mae Ploy bean stew sauce (Thai sweet hot sauce)
- 2 asparagus lances, slashed little
- 2 Tbsp green onion (scallions) slashed fine
- 2 Tbsp cilantro, slashed coarse (a major squeeze)
- 1 tsp five zest powder (clove, cinnamon, star anise, fennel seed, hua 'do pepper)

METHOD

1. Cook soba noodles for around 6 minutes (around 1 dime's breadth for each individual) then wash under cool water. While the noodle water is warming up in one pot, warm another pot with chicken stock, soy sauce, fish sauce, bean stew sauce, and 5-flavor. At the point when the stock achieves a bubble, place in the asparagus and turkey.
2. Stew until asparagus is simply mellowed. As the smoked turkey is as of now cooked, it simply needs to warm up and enhance the soup. Place 1/2 cup soba noodles in

every dish, Pour in 2 measures of stock alongside asparagus and turkey.
3. Top with sliced scallions and cilantro. This additionally tastes awesome with a few leaves of Thai basil and a sprinkle of zesty Sriracha bean stew sauce. It's a half breed of pho' style flavorings with Japanese style noodles. For a more real pho' you would utilize rice noodles with paper slim segments of hamburger flank on top.

13. Healthy Bean with Tofu, Peanut, and Broccoli

Ingredients

- 1/2 glass bean strings (1/2 ball saifun)
- 2 glasses chicken or vegetable stock (somewhat less if dishes are littler)
- 1/4 glass disintegrated dry shiitake mushrooms
- 1 Tbsp dried shrimp, slashed
- 4 oz. firm tofu (Chinese style)
- 1/8 glass cooked peanuts, smashed or slashed
- 1 little bloom of broccoli, broken into around 8 chomp size pieces
- 1 Tbsp soy sauce
- 1 Tbsp fish sauce
- 1/2 creep new ginger, ground
- sliced leaves of Thai basil, cilantro and parsley

Method

1. Spray the dried disintegrated shiitake mushrooms and sliced dried shrimp in warmed chicken (or vegetable) stock for 60 minutes, alongside the soy and fish sauce. No compelling reason to bubble yet, simply let the warm pot sit on the stove. Place dry saifun bean string in every serving dish. At the point when mushrooms in the pot of soup are delicate, heat another pot of plain water to the point of boiling and deliberately pour that hot plain water over the dry saifun in every dish. Let stand for around 10 minutes. Channel the unflavored water off the

INSULIN RESISTANCE

noodles before including the juices. This technique additionally serves to warm up the dishes so the soup stays hot longer at the table.

2. To complete the stock, add the ginger and tofu to the pot and expand heat until it bubbles. While that is warming up, steam the broccoli flowerettes in a secured dish in the microwave with a sprinkle of water and soy sauce, for around 2-3 minutes until delicate yet at the same time crunchy. You can likewise drop the brocoli in the juices for a couple of minutes, yet be mindful so as not to overcook it, or the juices will tackle a vegetal flavor. Mastermind the broccoli on top of the saifun noodles in every dish. Include the tofu and juices, then top with peanuts and crisp cleaved leaves of cilantro, Thai basil and parsley. Serve instantly.

14. Healthy Green Beans and Dumpling Soup

INGREDIENTS

- 4 oz. sushi grade ahi fish
- 1/2 tsp Sechuan pepper corns (hua 'do)
- 1/4 tsp salt
- 1 cup green beans (twelve or so crisp, or progressively if fancied)
- smashed garlic or shake of garlic powder
- sprinkle of soy sauce
- sprinkle of sesame oil
- 1 Tbsp smashed broiled peanuts
- 3 dumplings (see formula above)
- 1 cup soup (turkey, chicken, fish, and so forth.)
- 1 Tbsp shredded crisp ginger
- 1 squeeze Five Spice powder
- 1 Tbsp soy sauce

METHOD

1. slashed green onions, chives, cilantro, and so forth.

15. Healthy Salmon Burger

Ingredients

- 1/2 glass crude shrimp
- 3 protected artichoke hearts
- 1 glass crisp child spinach (compacted)
- 1 egg
- 1/4 expansive sweet onion
- 3 Tbsp green onion, slashed
- 1 tsp corn starch
- dash of salt

Method

1. Take after the dumpling formula above, with the egg wash, to make 20 or so dumplings. These will have a marginally more granular surface inside, due to some extent to the salmon. Flavors are more "green" and combine well with peas or greens like bok choy.
2. For the soup envisioned, heat two cups for each individual of turkey or chicken juices, include a dash of soy sauce, chile pieces, salt, fish sauce, 5-flavor and so on. Defrost 4-5 dumplings for each individual in the stock
3. . Just before serving, directly after the juices is bubbling once more, include 1/2 glass defrosted or crisp peas per individual and warmth just until bubbling once more. Include 1/2 to 1 measure of bean sprouts per individual and present with dumplings.

15. HEALTHY VEGETABLES WITH 3-BEAN SALAD

INGREDIENTS

- 1 substantial Chinese eggplant
- 1 medium zucchini (or two basic supply estimated little)
- 1-2 sweet red peppers
- 2 Tbsp olive oil
- squeeze of enhanced salt (sundried tomato salt for this situation)
- some slashed parsley and/or new basil
- balsamic vinegar – a sprinkle
- 1/2 glass three bean plate of mixed greens per individual.
- Prosciutto – a couple of shavings
- Shaved Parmesan – a sprinkle

METHOD

1. Cut the eggplant and zucchini the long way into long 1/8 creep thick cuts. Section the ringer peppers and expel the essence from inside, then cut into dainty strips. Brush everything daintily with olive oil and sprinkle with salt. Spread maybe a couple heating sheets with aluminum foil. Spread a meager film of olive oil on the foil. Turn on stove grill.
2. Orchestrate vegetables on the tray(s) with the goal that zucchini will hit the most sizzling spot in the oven. Put the eggplant and peppers close to the edge, or where they won't get the maxing out. Place sheets, each one in turn, under high warmth around 4 inches under the oven,

until tops begin to burn. Evacuate the main plate and embed the second (on the off chance that you are utilizing two) and watch nearly, as the second will go speedier. Expel the peppers from the plate, which have cooked on one side yet not the other (they are better less cooked.) Turn the majority of alternate vegetables so the uncooked sides face up, and put yet again under the grill until alternate sides are simply beginning to darken. Evacuate quickly. All out cooking time may be 4-10 minutes most extreme, contingent upon warmth.
3. Put all the vegetable on a platter in an enriching way. Sprinkle with balsamic vinegar, slashed basil or parsley and a touch of superb coarse salt. Serve promptly with some bean plate of mixed greens and other light accessories. I get a kick out of the chance to include a little measure of emphatically enhanced meat (incline prosciutto for instance) and a shaving of good matured parmesan cheddar to expand the flavors.
4. On the off chance that you are excessively ravenous, making it impossible to regard this as a fundamental course, it makes a decent canapé.

16. Amazing Lettuce Wrap Chicken

Ingredients

- 1 head margarine lettuce, entire clears out.
- 2-3 chicken thighs, boneless skinless, finely minced (4 oz. per individual)
- 1/2 sweet onion, slashed little
- 6 or so crisp catch mushrooms, sliced little (1-2 mugs)
- 2-3 glasses bean grows
- 1 glass sugar snap peas, sliced little
- 1/2 carrot, ground
- 1 celery stalk, finely slashed
- 1-2 green onions, slashed little
- 1/4 glasses broiled peanuts, pulverized
- 2 Tbsp hoisin sauce
- 1 Tbsp chinese rice cooking wine or mirin
- 1 Tbsp soy sauce
- 1 little clove garlic, squashed and minced
- 1 Tbsp sesame oil
- 1/4 glass sliced cilantro

Method

1. Separate the leaves of lettuce and clean them, then set them on a spotless towel to air dry while cooking. Hack the rest of the Ingredients and get them prepared close to the wok. Pre-heat the wok until smoking hot. Mix a dash of rice wine and soy sauce into a touch of hoisin sauce, alongside a touch of minced garlic, making the hoisin sufficiently runny to mix rapidly into the panfry toward the end.

INSULIN RESISTANCE

2. Brush the hot wok with bit of sesame oil, then include the minced chicken. Turn quickly for a couple of minutes, until generally cooked. Include the onions and mushrooms, and singe to expel some dampness, for a couple of more minutes. Hurl in the bean grows, minced pea pods, celery and shredded carrots, and mix quickly for one minute, to warm those Ingredients however not really to cook them. While mixing the new vegetables, hurl in the hoisin sauce blend, and expel from warmth when it is mixed in. Absolute cooking time shouldn't be more than around 5-6 minutes all the way.
3. Separate the panfry onto plates, and sprinkle with green onions, peanuts and cilantro before serving. Give a little bowl of additional hoisin sauce, to spread onto a lettuce leaf before filling the leaf with panfry, utilizing the lettuce as a wrapper to eat with hands.

17. Healthy Pumpkin Soup

Ingredients

- 5 glasses turkey stock
- 15 oz. pumpkin puree (1 can – don't utilize sweetened "pie filling")
- 15 oz. dark beans (1 can, or around 2 glasses)
- 2 onions, diced
- 1-2 red sweet peppers (relies on upon size)
- 1-2 canned chipotle peppers w/adobo sauce, minced
- 1 expansive clove garlic
- 2 Tbsp olive oil
- 2 tsp entire cumin, naturally ground
- 2 tsp smoked paprika (can substitute plain if distracted)
- 1 tsp salt – to taste
- 1 tsp mace or 1/2 tsp nutmeg
- 1 tsp sage
- 1 cup nonfat yogurt (or less relying upon surface)
- some cilantro and crisp tomato for embellishment

Method

1. Dice two onions and sweat them with 2 Tbsp olive oil and a dash of salt in a profound overwhelming soup pot, on medium low warmth, for around 30 minutes. They ought to be entirely soft at that point. It's OK on the off chance that they chestnut a bit, however blend regularly to ensure they don't blaze.
2. While the onions are sweating, utilize a couple of tongs to hold two entire new red ringer peppers over a high gas fire – or place them on a barbecue with high fire – and

INSULIN RESISTANCE

permit the fire to really smolder and darken the skin. You will hear sputtering and crackling. That is OK. Turn each moment or less, as they burn on every side, so the peppers get flared equitably. Expel from fire and put aside to cool. When you can deal with the peppers, cut them open and evacuate the seeds and substance. Hack coarsely.

3. Finely dice one huge garlic clove, and add the garlic to the mollified onions. Following a couple of minutes, include the turkey stock and raise the warmth a bit. (Chicken stock will do when there's no other option, yet keep an eye out for the salty sort, and lessen salt somewhere else as needs be. I make my own particular without salt.) After conveying the stock up to a low bubble, include a jar of pumpkin puree and a jar of dark beans (~1 3/4 mugs each). Include naturally ground cumin and sage, with some smoked paprika (if accessible) and a solid squeeze of mace or somewhat less of nutmeg. Mix in the flame broiled sliced ringer pepper.

4. Hack up maybe a couple canned chipotle peppers - the sort that comes wet in adobo sauce – and include the peppers with some of their sauce. These can get extremely hot, so alter amount to your sense of taste.

5. On the off chance that you don't have an inundation blender, the following stride requires that you take the pot off of the warmth and spoon the substance, in sensible parts, into a sustenance processor or blender. It's much simpler with a drenching blender, which culinary experts call a "giraffe", a handheld shaft with electric propeller toward the end which you can stick specifically into a pot of soup.

6. With the pot on low warmth or expelled from warmth, mix the substance with the electric blender while gradually including nonfat yogurt, one spoonful at once, holding up a minute as every expansion gets to be coordinated. Gradually mean a measure of yogurt, until the soup achieves a sought rich consistency.

7. Present with a sprinkle of cilantro and sliced tomatoes, or alongside a plate of mixed greens.

INSULIN RESISTANCE

18. Amazing Granola Muesli

INGREDIENTS

- 900 ml moved oats (325 g)
- 250 ml digestive wheat (45 g)
- 25 ml sunflower seeds (15 g)
- 25 ml linseed (15 g)
- 50 ml cashew nuts, slashed (30 g)
- 100 ml wholewheat flour (50 g)
- 50 ml nectar (discretionary)
- 15 ml canola oil
- 125 ml bubbling water
- 5 ml vanilla quintessence
- 125 ml raisins, sultanas or nutty cake blend (80 g)

METHOD

1. Blend the dry Ingredients. Bring the nectar, oil and water to the bubble. Include the warm fluid and enhancing to the dry Ingredients. Blend to shape a clammy blend and spread out onto a substantial preparing sheet.
2. Prepare at 150°C for 30 – 35 minutes. Blend the blend each 7 – 10 minutes, utilizing a fork, and separate huge bits of granola. Include raisins or dried foods grown from the ground well. Leave to cool. Store in a hermetically sealed compartment. Present with low-fat milk or yogurt, contingent upon inclination and eating routine solution.

19. Healthy Banana Breakfast Drink

Ingredients

- 30 ml Bokomo Fiber Plus or Kellogg's Hi-Fiber Bran breakfast oat (10 g)
- 50 ml bubbling water
- 1 firm, medium banana, cut into pieces (+-80 g peeled)
- 5 ml lemon juice
- 5 ml nectar (discretionary)
- 2 ml vanilla quintessence
- squeeze ground cinnamon
- 125 ml low-fat drain or plain low-fat yogurt

Method

1. Drench the breakfast grain in the bubbling water until the blend has chilled off. Put every one of the Ingredients in a liquidizer and liquidize until smooth and foamy. Serve instantly.
2. Apricot breakfast drink: Instead of banana, lemon squeeze and nectar, utilize 90 g Naturlite apricot parts and 15 ml depleted off apricot juice.

INSULIN RESISTANCE

20. Delicious Fried Chicken

Ingredients

- 100 ml olive oil
- 5 ml sliced garlic
- 3 medium leeks, washed and cut into rings (150 g)
- ½ medium red sweet pepper, seeded and cut into strips (75 g)
- ½ medium green sweet pepper, seeded and cut into strips (75 g)
- 100 g new mushrooms, cut
- 500 g chicken filets, cut into strips
- 1 medium pineapple, peeled, cored and cubed (350 g)
- 25 ml chestnut onion soup powder
- 25 ml cornflour
- 25 ml soy sauce
- 50 ml water
- 250 ml bubbling water

Method

1. Heat the oil and panfry the garlic, leeks, sweet peppers and mushrooms until the mushrooms are cooked. Add the chicken strips to the vegetable blend and panfry until the meat changes shading and is cooked.
2. Blend in the pineapple solid shapes and panfry until simply cooked. Blend the soup powder and cornflour with the soy sauce and water until smooth. Blend the bubbling water into the glue and add the subsequent soup blend to the seared blend. Cook, blending, for 1 minute, until the sauce thickens and is cooked.

21. Amazing Moussaka

Ingredients

- 1 medium brinjal (+-350 g)
- 5 ml olive oil
- 5 ml cleaved garlic
- 1 substantial onion, peeled and slashed (150 g)
- 500 g incline meat mince
- ½ meat stock shape, disintegrated
- 125 ml bubbling water
- 25 ml tomato glue
- 10 ml dried parsley
- 5 ml dried blended herbs
- 2 ml ground cinnamon
- crisply ground dark pepper
- 1 ml salt (discretionary)

Cheddar Sauce:
- 60 ml cake flour
- 400 ml low-fat milk
- 2 ml salt
- squeeze pepper
- 1 ml ground nutmeg
- 1 medium egg, beaten (50 g)
- 125 ml ground Tussers cheddar (50 g)
- paprika

Method

INSULIN RESISTANCE

1. Cut the unpeeled brinjal into 5 mm thick cuts. Absorb salted water for 30 minutes. Deplete and wash in frosty water. Bubble for 3 to 5 minutes in a little water until the brinjal is cooked yet at the same time firm.
2. Heat the oil and panfry the garlic and onion until the onion is translucent. Add the mince to the broiled blend and panfry until the meat is light cocoa. Mix the rest of the Ingredients, aside from the brace, into the meat blend. Taste and add salt to taste. Orchestrate a large portion of the brinjal cuts in a solitary layer in an elongated ovenproof dish. Spoon the meat blend over the brinjal and spread out uniformly. Orchestrate the rest of the brinjal cuts over the meat. Pour the cheddar sauce over and sprinkle the rest of the cheddar and paprika over the dish. Heat at 180°C for 35 to 40 minutes. Serve hot with rice and a fresh plate of mixed greens. On the off chance that your dietary medicine permits more sugars, you may add a whole wheat bread move to the feast.
3. Cheddar Sauce:
4. Blend the flour and a little drain until smooth. Convey the rest of the milk to the bubble. Stream the flour glue into the bubbling milk, mixing constantly. Cook, blending for 2 – 3 minutes, until the sauce as thickened and is cooked. Season the sauce with sat, pepper and nutmeg. Mix the egg and a large portion of the cheddar into the white sauce.

22. Tasty Lentil Sauce

INGREDIENTS

- 275 ml dried chestnut lentils (220 g)
- 500 ml water
- 1 straight leaf
- squeeze ground cloves
- squeeze naturally ground dark pepper, or to taste
- 30 ml olive oil
- 2 medium onions, peeled and slashed (200 g)
- 2 celery stalks and leaves, slashed (25 g)
- 125 g white catch mushrooms, cut
- 50 ml tomato purée
- 600 ml hot vegetable concentrate or 10 ml Marmite broke up in 60 ml bubbling water
- 50 ml vinegar
- 1 medium green apple, peeled, cored, ground (100 g)
- 50 ml sliced new parsley
- salt and pepper to taste

METHOD

1. Spray the lentils for 2 hours in water to cover. Channel. Place the lentils, 500 ml water, the inlet leaf, cloves and dark pepper in a pan. Stew over low warmth until the lentils are delicate and cooked (30 to 40 minutes). Channel.
2. Heat the oil and panfry the onions and garlic until the onions are translucent. Include the carrots, celery and mushrooms to the onions and panfry until the vegetables are cooked yet at the same time fresh delicate.

INSULIN RESISTANCE

3. Blend the cooked lentils in the vegetable blend. Blend the tomato purée, vegetable concentrate and vinegar and mix into the lentil blend with the apple. Stew for 30 to 4 minutes, until the sauce is flavorsome and cooked.
4. Mix the slashed parsley into the sauce and season with salt and pepper to taste. Serve hot on cooked pasta. Include a fresh plate of mixed greens as wanted, contingent upon dietary rules.

23. Healthy Potato and Carrot Bake

Ingredients

- 5 – 6 medium sweet potatoes, unpeeled, cut into 5 mm thick cuts (500 g)
- 2 - 3 medium carrots, peeled and coarsely ground (225 g)
- 1 substantial Granny Smith apple, cored, peeled and cut into cuts (150 g)
- 50 ml cleaved crisp parsley
- 1 ml salt
- crisply ground pepper to taste
- 125 ml cheddar, ground (50 g)
- 250 ml low-fat milk
- 2 medium eggs, beaten (100 g)
- ground nutmeg

Method

1. Heat up the sweet potatoes for 15 minutes in a little water, until simply cooked. Channel. Steam the ground carrots of 5 to 10 minutes, until simply cooked, and still fresh.
2. Layer the Ingredients in a lubed 250 mm x 250 mm ovenproof dish as takes after: a large portion of the sweet potato cuts, carrots, apple, parsley, salt, pepper and cheddar. Rehash the layers.
3. Beat together the milk and egg and pour over the dish. Sprinkle nutmeg on top and cover the dish with a top or

INSULIN RESISTANCE

thwart. Heat for 20 minutes at 180°C. Evacuate the cover and prepare for a further 25 to 30 minutes, until the egg blend has set. Serve hot, with a fundamental dish, for example, broil chicken.

24. Healthy Apple and Raisin Cake

Ingredients

- 250 ml wholewheat flour (130 g)
- 250 ml cake flour (120 g)
- 2 ml salt
- 5 ml blended zest
- 5 ml heating powder
- 125 ml fructose (100 g)
- 125 ml seedless raisins (75 g)
- 2 substantial apples, peeled and ground (200 g ground)
- 5 ml bicarbonate of pop
- 250 ml buttermilk
- 2 medium eggs, beaten (100 g)
- 50 ml canola oil
- ground cinnamon

Method

1. Blend the dry Ingredients and mix the raisins and ground apple into the blend. Beat the bicarbonate of pop, buttermilk, eggs and oil together. Blend the milk blend into the dry Ingredients. Mix until simply blended.
2. Spoon the player into a lubed 230 mm x 230 mm cake dish and level the surface. Sprinkle cinnamon over the player. Prepare for 35 to 40 minutes at 180°C until brilliant chestnut and cooked. Permit to cool in the cake prospect minutes, then turn out onto a wire cooling rack to cool totally.
3. Remark: Apple and raisin cake tastes best naturally prepared, however keeps well in the cooler for up to five

INSULIN RESISTANCE

days. Warm the bars of apple and raisin cake for 15 to 20 seconds in the microwave before serving. The bars can be solidified.

25. Tasty Sweet Potato and Date Cake

Ingredients

- 200 ml dates, finely slashed (125 g)
- 125 ml bubbling water
- 5 ml bicarbonate of pop
- 1 medium sweet potato, peeled and ground (200 g)
- 1 expansive Granny Smith apple, peeled and ground (100 g)
- 2 expansive eggs, beaten (110 g)
- 125 ml buttermilk
- 50 ml immaculate nectar
- 50 ml canola oil
- 250 ml whole wheat flour (130 g)
- 250 ml cake flour (120 g)
- 2 ml salt
- 5 ml ground cinnamon
- 5 ml ground nutmeg
- 5 ml preparing powder

Method

1. Place the dates in an extensive blending dish and pour the bubbling water over them. Sprinkle the bicarbonate of pop over the dates and blend to blend. Put aside to cool. Blend the sweet potato, apple, eggs, drain, nectar and oil into the cooled date blend. Blend the dry Ingredients, lifting the blend with the spoon as you work, keeping in mind the end goal to consolidate air.

INSULIN RESISTANCE

2. Include the dates and sweet potato blend to the dry Ingredients and blend to create a sticky mixture. Spoon the mixture into a lubed 250 mm x 250 mm cake skillet. Level the surface of the player.
3. Prepare for 50 to a hour at 180°C until brilliant cocoa and cooked. Embed a stick in the focal point of the blend to test whether it is finished.
4. Turn the cake out onto a wire cooling rack to cool totally. Cut the cake into bars and store in a sealed shut compartment.

26. Pasta with Lentil Marinara Sauce

Ingredients

- 1 pound pasta of decision
- 1 cup (26 ounces) without fat low-sodium tomato-based pasta sauce
- 1 can (15 ounces) lentils, washed and depleted
- 1/2 cup dry red wine (can be nonalcoholic) or low-sodium veggie lover soup
- Salt to taste
- Crisply ground dark pepper

Method

1. Cook the pasta as indicated by bundle Method.
2. In the mean time, consolidate the pasta sauce, lentils, and wine or stock in a medium pot. Warm delicately and season with the salt and pepper. Serve over the depleted pasta.

27. HEALTHY CHERRY TOMATO AND BROWN RICE SALAD WITH ARTICHOKE HEARTS

INGREDIENTS

- 3 mugs warm chestnut basmati rice
- 6 ounces marinated artichoke hearts, flushed in heated water, depleted, and cut
- 1 glass sliced scallions
- 1/2 pounds red, yellow, or blended cherry tomatoes, divided
- 1/2 glass sliced new basil
- 1/2 glass without fat Italian dressing
- 3 tablespoons lemon juice
- 2 cloves garlic, pounded
- 1/4 teaspoon salt
- Crisply ground dark pepper to taste
- 1 head fresh lettuce

METHOD

1. Place the rice in an extensive plate of mixed greens bowl and include the artichoke hearts, scallions, tomatoes, and basil. Blend delicately. Join the Italian dressing, lemon juice, garlic, salt, and pepper in a little bowl or cup.
2. Whisk or shake until all around mixed. Pour over the plate of mixed greens and blend delicately. Serve on beds of lettuce on individual plates.

28. Berry Mousse

INGREDIENTS

- 1 bundle (12.3 ounces) lessened fat additional firm smooth tofu, disintegrated
- 2 3/4 glasses defrosted solidified unsweetened berries of decision
- 3 tablespoons sugar or 2 tablespoons agave nectar
- 1 tablespoon berry alcohol (discretionary)

METHOD

1. Mix the tofu, berries, sugar or agave nectar, and alcohol, if utilizing, in a blender or sustenance processor until smooth. Spoon into 4 pudding dishes and refrigerate until chilled.

INSULIN RESISTANCE

29. BLOOD SUGAR BALANCER

INGREDIENTS

- 2 cucumbers
- 5-6 stalks celery
- ½ zucchini
- ¼ bundle Kale with stems (my most loved is Lacinato, yet any will do)
- parsley
- 2-3 leaves of dandelion greens
- 1 lemon
- 1-2 green apples (discretionary)
- 1 ½ inch handle new ginger root
- ½ finger of turmeric

METHOD

1. Wash and prepare all Ingredients; squeeze and appreciate!

30. HEALTHY MEAL

INGREDIENTS

- 1-1/some non-dairy milk.
- Eden Extra Plain Soymilk
- 3 tablespoons of chia seeds
- 1 ready (dotted) banana
- 2-3 set dates (can include 1-2 parcels of stevia on the off chance that you need a sweeter pudding)
- 1-15 ounce jar of 100% Pumpkin (like Libby's)
- 2 teaspoons vanilla
- 2 teaspoons cinnamon
- 1/2 to 3/4 teaspoon of nutmeg
- raisins and toasted walnuts to sprinkle on top of individual servings.

METHOD

1. Add the crude groats to vast dish, and absorb 4 some water. I let them douse overnight, yet they have to spray for 60 minutes, least. Overnight drenching is simple.
2. In the wake of dousing, wash well two or three times to expel the coagulated covering.
3. The first 2 measures of drenched groats grow to 4 mugs. Hold 1 cup to add back to the last pudding toward the end.
4. Include the washed groats, short the saved glass, the "milk", the chia, the pumpkin, the banana, the dates, the vanilla, the cinnamon, and the nutmeg to a blender or processor. I utilize a VitaMix. Mix well.
5. Taste, include a little stevia is you need a sweeter taste.

INSULIN RESISTANCE

6. Empty everything into a substantial dish, then blend in the held measure of entire groats. This gives it a pleasant nutty crunchy taste and composition without the calories of nuts.
7. Trim 1 glass servings with a couple of raisins and toasted walnuts.
8. Refrigerate the scraps and appreciate 5 days of buckwheat breakfast pudding.

30. Tasty Chipotle Cashew Topping

Ingredients

- 1/some crude cashews absorbed 1/some water for 60 minutes. Longer is fine.
- 3-4 tablespoons of crisply crushed lime juice
- 2 coarsely cleaved garlic cloves, less to taste
- 1/2 to 1 canned chipotle pepper in adobo sauce. Sizes shift, so go gradually - you can simply include more
- a couple grains of coarse ocean salt to taste

Method

1. Drench the crude cashews for no less than one hour in 1/some water
2. Into a force blender (VitaMix works best) include the cashews AND the drenching water, the garlic, the lime juice, and the chipotle.
3. Mix well until the cashews are a smooth, satiny consistency. Check for taste. Include more chipotle, in the event that you like.
4. Include a couple grains of salt to taste.

31. Tasty Creamy Chipotle Chia

INGREDIENTS

- 1/some Eden Extra Plain Soymilk (wealthier than other non-dairy milks)
- 3 tablespoons of newly pressed lime juice
- 2 coarsely sliced garlic cloves, less to taste
- 1/2 to 1 canned chipotle pepper in adobo sauce. Sizes differ, so go moderate - you can simply include more
- 3 tablespoons of white chia (I like the Salba brand)
- 1 teaspoon of agave (more to taste, if necessary)
- a couple grains of coarse ocean salt

METHOD

1. Include every one of the Ingredients into a force blender (I utilize a VitaMix), including the chia seed just before you're prepared to turn the blender on.
2. Mix well, until the consistency is smooth and plush.
3. Taste, and include additional chipotle, salt, or agave to your own particular taste.

32. Tasty Smoked Salmon Wraps

Ingredients

- 5 delicate tortilla wraps
- 250g smooth low-fat curds
- 1 ml ground lemon skin
- 25ml new lemon juice
- 5ml finely sliced onion
- 25ml tricks
- 25ml sliced crisp parsley or fennel
- 200g smoked snoek

Method

1. To make the tortillas less demanding to move up, warmth them in the microwave stove for a few moments, or wrap them in foil and warmth in a preheated broiler for a couple of minutes. Meanwhile, join the curds, lemon skin, juice and onion.
2. Spoon around 50ml of the curds blend onto a tortilla and spread to around 2cm from the edge. Sprinkle the tricks and parsley over the blend and place the smoked salmon on top. Fold two sides of the tortilla over to within and move up as you would a flapjack. Sliced down the middle and serve.

INSULIN RESISTANCE

33. Amazing Sweet Potato Muffins

Ingredients

- 200g peeled sweet potato, cut
- 1 medium apple, peeled, cored and cut (100g peeled)
- 350ml Sasko wheat rich Self-raising flour (175g) or high-fiber self-raising flour
- 100ml oat wheat (70g)
- 1.25ml salt
- 25g pecan nuts, cleaved
- 50ml currants (30g)
- 10ml finely ground orange skin
- 75ml crisp squeezed orange
- 50ml sunflower oil
- 75ml immaculate crude nectar
- 125ml low-fat buttermilk
- 2 vast eggs, isolated
- 5ml vanilla quintessence
- 2.5ml bicarbonate of pop

Method

1. Cook the sweet potato and apple in a little water until delicate and done. Deplete, squash and put aside to cool. Combine the flour, oat wheat, salt, nuts, currants and orange skin. Include the squeezed orange, oil, nectar, buttermilk, egg yolk, vanilla pith and bicarbonate of pop to the sweet potato blend and blend.
2. Blend the sweet potato blend into the dry Ingredients. Beat the egg whites until hardened and overlap into the mixture. Spoon the mixture into a lubed 18-glass biscuit

KATYA JOHANSSON

tin. Prepare in a pre-warmed stove at 180°C for 30 to 35 minutes until brilliant cocoa and done.

INSULIN RESISTANCE

34. AMAZING CRUMPETS

INGREDIENTS

- 250ml Sasko grain rich self-raising flour (130g)
- 125ml Whole wheat Pronutro
- 5ml preparing powder
- 1.25ml salt
- 10ml oil, for example, macadamia nut oil
- 1 substantial egg
- 350ml low-fat milk

METHOD

1. Consolidate the flour, Pronutro, heating powder and salt. Beat the oil, egg and drain together. Add the milk blend to the dry Ingredients and race with an inflatable speed until smooth. Heat a skillet until medium hot.
2. Shower with non-stick sustenance spray or utilize a paper towel to wipe a little oil over the surface of the skillet. Spoon 50ml hitter into the griddle for every crumpet, ensuring they are adequately far separated.
3. Permit space for the hitter to rise and spread. Cook the crumpets until air pockets show up at first glance and start to break. Turn with an egg lifter and cook until brilliant on both sides. Place the crumpets on a wire rack and cover with a spotless tea towel to keep them from drying out while the rest are made.

35. Healthy Berry Yogurt Mousse

Ingredients

- 300 ml Flavored low fat yogurt (Hijke or Woolworths)
- 300 g puréed strawberries/different berries
- 60 ml Apple Juice/Water
- 10 g gelatine
- 2 egg whites raced till hardened
- 50 g caster sugar
- 250 ml cream, whipped

Method

1. In a pan, warmth the squeezed apple yet don't bubble. Expel from warmth and Sprinkle the gelatine at first glance. Delicately blend to break up. Leave to remain to cool to room temperature.
2. Whisk egg whites. Also, crease in the castor sugar. Whisk cream.. Fold the gelatine into the pureed natural product. Crease together everything except the cream and overlap this in last. Empty into 125 ml ramekins or little glasses. Chill for 2 hours and serve finished with berries

36. Creamy Tomato Soup

INGREDIENTS

- 15 medium estimated tomatoes (around 1,2 kg)
- '3 sweet red peppers or 2 red one and 1 yellow one in the event that you purchase a blended bundle
- ½ cup dairy cream or coconut cream
- ¼ cup olive oil
- 3 huge sprigs of rosemary
- 6 huge cloves of garlic
- 1 liter of value vegetable or chicken stock (Ready made is alright given it doesn't contain hydrogenated fat).
- 2 tablespoons tomato puree
- Salt and dark pepper to taste.
- 1 – 2 tbs (15-30 ml) of sugar (discretionary)

METHOD

1. Preheat broiler to 180 degrees.
2. Cut the tomatoes in quarters.
3. Remove the pips from the sweet peppers and cut them in quarters too.
4. Expel the external layer from the garlic cloves.
5. Place the tomatoes, peppers, garlic and rosemary twigs on a preparing plate and sprinkle with the olive oil. Utilize your hands to guarantee that the vegetables are well secured.
6. Prepare for 30 – 45 minutes amidst the stove till the peppers are all around cooked. The tomatoes will gaze very withered upward at this point.

7. Expel the preparing plate from the broiler and leave to cook somewhat so you can deal with the sprigs of rosemary. Expel the leaves utilizing your fingers and dispose of the stick – however not the takes off.
8. Include every one of the vegetables and herbs and broiled garlic to an expansive bowl or pot. Utilize a portion of the stock to mix the vegetables to a smooth puree. Presently include whatever is left of the stock and cream or coconut cream.
9. Include salt, pepper and sugar to taste at this stage. Warm in the pot or in a microwaveable dish when you are prepared to serve. Present with crisp coriander or basil.

37. Tasty Tomato Sauce

Ingredients

- 2 measures of diced onions
- 3 cloves of garlic (minced)
- 2 x 400g tins of smashed tomatoes
- 1-2 tablespoons of dried basil
- 1/2 teaspoon of dried rosemary
- 2 tablespoons coconut oil
- 1/4 teaspoon of celery seed
- 4 inlet leaves (expel in the wake of cooking)
- 3-4 tablespoons of dried thyme
- 2 tablespoons of dried marjoram
- 2 tablespoons of dried parsley
- 1 stick of cinnamon
- celery takes off
- salt to taste

Method

1. Heat the oil in a huge dish utilizing a medium-high warmth. Include the onions and cook for 5 minutes blending regularly. At that point add the garlic and keep on stirring for another 2-3 minutes.
2. Add the rest of the Ingredients and stew on low warmth revealed until the sauce starts to thicken (roughly 20 minutes).
3. Once the fancied consistency has been accomplished expel the sauce from the warmth and permit to cool. After it has cooled evacuate the cove leaves and cinnamon stick.

KATYA JOHANSSON

4. Place in clear glass jugs or other fixed holders.

38. Tasty Grill Sauce

Ingredients

- 1 glass apple juice vinegar
- 1 tin of pounded tomatoes
- 1 onion (cleaved up)
- 4 cloves of garlic (minced)
- 2 tablespoons coconut oil
- 2 tablespoons of mustard seeds
- 1 tablespoon Worcestershire sauce
- 1 cove leaf
- 1 tablespoon bean stew powder
- 2 teaspoons dried sage
- 2 teaspoons dried thyme
- 1 teaspoon salt
- 1 teaspoon dark pepper
- 1 stick of cinnamon
- 1/2 glass water

Method

1. Heat the coconut oil in an expansive skillet utilizing a medium-high warmth. Include the onions and cook for 5 minutes blending frequently. At that point add the garlic and keep on stirring for another 2-3 minutes.
2. Add the rest of the Ingredients (vinegar keep going) and stew on low warmth revealed until the sauce starts to thicken (around 20 minutes).
3. Once the craved consistency has been accomplished expel the sauce from the warmth and permit to cool.

KATYA JOHANSSON

   After it has cooled expel the cove leaves and cinnamon stick.
4. Place in clear glass jugs or other fixed holders.

INSULIN RESISTANCE

39. TASTY CURRIED CARROT SOUP

INGREDIENTS

- 1 tablespoon olive oil
- 1 teaspoon mustard seed
- 1/2 yellow onion, cleaved
- 1 pound carrots, peeled and cut into 1/2-inch pieces
- 1 tablespoon in addition to 1 teaspoon peeled and cleaved crisp ginger
- 1/2 jalapeno bean stew, seeded
- 2 teaspoons curry powder
- 5 mugs chicken stock, vegetable stock or juices
- 1/4 glass cleaved crisp cilantro (new coriander), in addition to leaves for enhancement
- 2 tablespoons crisp lime juice
- 1/2 teaspoon salt (discretionary)
- 3 tablespoons low-fat acrid cream or sans fat plain yogurt
- Ground pizzazz of 1 lime

METHOD

1. In a substantial pan, warm the olive oil over medium warmth. Include the mustard seed. At the point when the seeds simply begin to pop, after around 1 minute, include the onion and saute until delicate and translucent, around 4 minutes. Include the carrots, ginger, jalapeno and curry powder and saute until the seasonings are fragrant, around 3 minutes.
2. Include 3 measures of the stock, raise the warmth to high and heat to the point of boiling. Decrease the

warmth to medium-low and stew, revealed, until the carrots are delicate, around 6 minutes.
3. In a blender or nourishment processor, puree the soup in groups until smooth and come back to the pot. Mix in the rest of the 2 cups stock. Return the soup to medium warmth and warm tenderly. Just before serving, blend in the cleaved cilantro and lime juice. Season with the salt, if wanted.
4. Scoop into warmed individual dishes. Trim with a shower of yogurt, a sprinkle of lime pizzazz and cilantro clears out.

40. Amazing Red Tomato Salsa

Ingredients

- 4 medium tomatoes
- 1 little pack of scallions
- ½ c. cilantro
- ½ jalapeno
- ¼ tsp cumin
- ½ lemon
- Salt

Method

1. A large portion of the tomatoes and press out the majority of the juice and seeds in the waste. Hack the tomatoes into eighths (major pieces). Add to nourishment processor. Finely slash scallions, jalapeno, and cilantro; add to the tomatoes. Crush in the juice of the lemon. Sprinkle in the cumin and include a squeeze of salt.
2. Beat the sustenance processor four or five times, sufficiently only to blend well and separate the tomatoes more – making them succulent yet at the same time stout. In the event that you like a "smooth" salsa, mix until you achieve the consistency you lean toward.

41. Green Smoothie

Ingredients

- 6   fl oz unsweetened almond milk
- 1/3   banana
- 1/2   cup pineapple, crisp or solidified
- tbsp almond or nutty spread
- Medjool dates, set
- tsp ground cinnamon
- glasses spinach, stuffed
- glass ice 3D shapes

Method

1. Add Ingredients to FourSide or WildSide+ jug all together recorded and secure top. Select "Smoothie" and appreciate.

INSULIN RESISTANCE

42. Tasty Chicken, Mushroom and Porcini Soup Recipe

Ingredients

- measures of arranged vegetable stock
- 100 g incline chicken bosom
- ½ carrot, diced
- ¼ leek, cut thick
- mushrooms, cut slim
- little bits of dried porcini
- cleaved parsley for enhancement

Method

1. In a pot, convey the vegetable stock to bubble.
2. Include chicken bosom and when it's cooked through, evacuate and put aside.
3. Add the vegetables to the stock.
4. Utilizing two forks, shred the chicken into slight pieces then add to the vegetables and stock.
5. The soup is prepared when the carrots are done yet at the same time somewhat firm to the nibble.
6. Present with cleaved parsley.

KATYA JOHANSSON

43. Healthy Broccoli and Turmeric Soup

Ingredients

little head of broccoli, cut into florets
- ½ onion, slashed
- 1 garlic, cut
- ½ celery stalk, slashed
- ½ teaspoon of turmeric
- ¼ teaspoon ground ginger
- 1 bayleaf
- entire dark peppercorns
- vegetable stock or Massel vegetable block with water

Method

1. Include every single arranged vegetable and flavors to a microwave safe dish.
2. Add enough stock just to cover.
3. Cook in the microwave for 15 minutes on high.
4. When it has chilled off, procedure with a blender stick.

INSULIN RESISTANCE

44. Tasty Chicken and Vegetable Zoodle Soup

Ingredients

- measures of arranged vegetable stock
- ¼ cup shredded poached chicken
- carrots, diced
- 1 zucchini, julienned
- mushrooms, cut
- bunch Cauliflower florets
- bunch Broccoli florets
- inch Leek, daintily cut
- 1 celery, stalk, cleaved
- 1 squash, cleaved
- Modest bunch of child spinach clears out

Method

1. In a pot, convey stock to the bubble. Include vegetables and cook for 5 to 10 minutes until only delicate.

45. Tasty Sushi Roll Recipe

Ingredients

- cup cauliflower rice
- tablespoons of rice vinegar
- crisply ground ginger
- nori sheets
- can fish in saline solution
- long shallot, cut thin longwise
- modest bunch of coriander
- soy sauce for plunging

Method

1. Get ready cauliflower rice.
2. Heat a non stick cup and toast the cauliflower rice until marginally brilliant.
3. Include a little rice vinegar and ground ginger and give it a decent blend. Put aside to cool.
4. On a sushi mat, lay the nori sheet unpleasant side up.
5. Include the cauliflower rice, leaving around 2 cm every side.
6. Include a slight line of wasabi over the rice.
7. Top with depleted canned fish, cut shallots and coriander.
8. Move into a sushi roll.
9. Utilizing a sharp blade, cut the move into nibble measured bits of fifty-fifty askew.
10. Present with soy sauce.

46. Healthy Wholesome Vegetable Stock

Ingredients

- carrot, hacked
- little onion, hacked
- 1 huge garlic clove, meagerly cut
- 4 mushrooms, daintily cut
- modest bunch of parsley stalks
- 1 leek, white separated just washed and cut
- 1 bayleaf
- 4 entire dark peppercorns
- squeezes of ocean salt
- 1 sprig of rosemary
- water

Method

1. In a huge pot, include every one of the vegetables the add water to fill the pot.
2. Convey to the bubble then stew for 20 minutes.
3. Go through a strainer and dispose of the solids.
4. In the event that you wish, you can run the stock through a muslin material.
5. Store in the refrigerator or partition into bits and store in the cooler.

47. Tasty Turmeric Tea Golden Milk Recipe

INGREDIENTS

- ¼ glass coconut milk
- ¼ teaspoon of turmeric
- ⅛ teaspoon of cinnamon
- spot of broke dark pepper

METHOD

1. Blend all fixings in an espresso mug.
2. Delicately warm in the microwave until warm yet don't give it a chance to bubble, roughly 40 seconds.
3. Serve in a coffee mug.

INSULIN RESISTANCE

48. Tasty Burrata with Rocket and Cherry Tomatoes

Ingredients

- burrata
- measures of child rocket clears out
- ½ punnet of cooked cherry tomatoes
- Salt and pepper
- teaspoon of olive oil

Method

1. Lay the rocket leaves on a plate. Include the burrata in the middle. Include cherry tomatoes the outside.
2. Shower with a little,olive oil.
3. Season with salt and pepper.

49. Tasty Basturma Egg Cups

Ingredients

- eggs
- 5 meager cuts of basturma

Method

1. Preheat a fan constrained broiler to 160C.
2. Utilizing 2 basturma cuts, line silicone mold biscuit tin to shape a cross example.
3. Technique 1 - delicately soften an entire egg up the biscuit cup.
4. Technique 2 - cut the rest of the cut of basturma into little pieces. In a little bowl, whisk the egg with the bits of basturma then tenderly fill lined biscuit skillet.
5. Heat for roughly 10-15 minutes relying upon how you like your eggs.
6. Present with rocket serving of mixed greens.

50. Tasty Zucchini and Squash Bake

Ingredients

- zucchinis, meagerly cut
- squash, cut down the middle then daintily cut
- clove garlic, minced
- sprigs of Fresh thyme
- tablespoons of olive oil
- ¼ cup shaved Parmesan cheddar

Method

1. Set up the vegetables then place then in a level preparing dish.
2. Include the minced garlic and thyme.
3. Include the olive oil and blend well.
4. Top with shaved Parmesan cheddar.
5. Prepare in 160C fan constrained broiler for 20 minutes on until fresh and the cheddar has softened.
6. Serve as a side dish.

KATYA JOHANSSON

PLANT BASED DIET COOKBOOK:

50 Plant Based Recipes (Breakfast, Lunch, Dinner & Dressings) For Anyone Who's On A Healthy Plant Based Nutrition Lifestyle

KATYA JOHANSSON

Copyright © 2016. All Rights Reserved.

INSULIN RESISTANCE

INTRODUCTION

Plant-based cooking doesn't need to exhaust or comprise just of servings of mixed greens, fluid suppers and dull steamed vegetables. There are a lot of worldwide food impacts, from Asian to Mediterranean, that component a variety of supplement thick plants cooked in fragrant herbs and stacked with restorative properties that make dishes luscious.

Incorporating plant sustenance like mushrooms and beans as the point of convergence of a supper instead of chicken or hamburger is the best and most straightforward approach to begin. Pick a fixing and manufacture out by picking reciprocal vegetables and flavors.

Battles like Meatless Mondays commit a whole day to sans meat eating. Setting aside a few minutes for cooking is just about as critical as choosing what to eat. Basic, at-home and produced using scratch cooking will transform dietary patterns into a way of life. In the event that your timetable doesn't allow a minute ago sustenance choices, ensure you feast Method for the week.

KATYA JOHANSSON

INSULIN RESISTANCE

BREAKFAST RECIPES

1. HEALTHY PUMPKIN PANCAKES

INGREDIENTS

- 1/2 glass oats
- 1/4 glass cornmeal
- 1/4 glass entire wheat flour *Gluten-Free form
- 2 t. preparing powder
- 1 t. preparing pop
- 1/2 t. salt
- 1/2 cup pumpkin puree (canned) *
- 1 t. ground cinnamon
- 1/2 t. ground ginger
- 1/2 t. allspice
- 1 t. vanilla concentrate
- 1 huge or 2 little ready banana, pounded
- 1/2 cup non-dairy milk

METHOD

1. Preheat frying pan to medium.
2. Put the greater part of the dry Ingredients in an big bowl and mix to join.
3. Blend the wet Ingredients, banana, pumpkin, vanilla, and non-dairy milk, in a different bowl and whisk.
4. Consolidate the wet and dry Ingredients until simply wet.

KATYA JOHANSSON

5. Delicately shower your iron with oil and drop the hitter by big spoonful onto it. Cook until air pockets begin to conform to the edges and the base is pleasantly sautéed.
6. Flip and cook the other side.
7. Present with maple syrup or jam and your most loved products of the soil or nuts.

INSULIN RESISTANCE

2. Healthy Groovy Green Smoothie

Ingredients

- 1 glass natural berries
- 1 orange peeled into areas
- 3 romaine lettuce clears out
- 3/4 glass almond milk
- 1/2 scoop Super Seed

Method:

1. Placed all into blender aside from the Super Seed.
2. Mix until smooth. Include a little water if too thick.
3. Pour in the Super Seed and buzz only a few moments.

3. Amazing Tofu Scramble

Ingredients

- 1 bundle firm tofu, depleted and disintegrated
- 1 onion, generally cleaved
- 1 red pepper, generally cleaved
- 1/2 to 1 8 oz. cup mushrooms, cut
- 1/2 tsp. turmeric
- 1/2 tsp curry power
- Salt and pepper to taste

Method

1. Saute the greater part of the vegetables in a little measure of water in non-stick dish.
2. At the point when veggies are for the most part delicate, include the disintegrated tofu, flavors and salt and pepper and mix to join. The blend ought to turn yellow from the flavors and start to look like eggs.
3. Keep on cooking until the vast majority of dampness from the tofu has cooked off and it's warmed through, blending much of the time so as not to stick.

INSULIN RESISTANCE

4. Amazing Potato Pancakes

Ingredients

- 2 glasses pureed potatoes
- 1/4 minced onion (or ground)
- Include around 1 tsp. of any herbs or flavors you like, for example, parsley, chives, or curry.
- 1/4 Flour (use anything you have, oat, entire wheat, buckwheat...)
- Salt and pepper to taste

Method

1. Blend the majority of the Ingredients in an extensive dish.
2. Heat an big skillet and utilize a little oil or spray to avert staying. A non-stick cup truly makes a difference.
3. Drop by vast spoonful onto the hot skillet and spread a little with your spoon and fingers.
4. Flip when cooked on one side (around 2-3 min.)
5. Level more with you spatula and cook until sautéed on the second side.
6. Present with fruit purée, maple syrup or blueberries.

5. Delicious Soy Yogurt

Ingredients

- 3 Tblsp. cornstarch
- 1 box of normal or unsweetened soy milk (not chilled).
- 1-2 Tblsp. sugar or maple syrup
- Sweet thermometer
- Yogurt Starter

Method:

1. Include some soy milk to a pan and begin warming.
2. Pour 1/some icy soy milk into a measuring glass and speed in 3 Tbl. cornstarch.
3. Once the milk in the pot begins to steam, speed in the cornstarch blend. Proceed to warmth and race until it begins to thicken.
4. Expel from the warmth. Speed in whatever is left of the soy drain and let the temperature come down to no less than 110 degrees F.
5. Rush in the starter to mix and fill the holders.
6. Take after the guideline on your yogurt producer for time.

INSULIN RESISTANCE

6. AMAZING POWER PORRIDGE

INGREDIENTS

- 2 cups almond or oat milk
- 1 T. lentils
- 2 T. steel cut oats
- 2 T. oat grain
- 1 T. Kasha (buckwheat groats, toasted)
- 1 T. flax seeds, ground
- 1 T. chia seeds
- 1 T. sunflower seeds
- 2 T. walnuts, harsh cleaved
- 1 T. pumpkin seeds, crude
- 4 huge dates, harsh cleaved
- 1 T. raisins
- new or solidified berries and/or bananas

METHOD:

1. Heat almond or oat milk to a bubble include lentils, then include grains, seeds and oats mix, turn down the warmth to stew, mixing sometimes. Stew for around fifteen minutes until the lentils are delicate. You may need to add more almond milk to keep the consistency smooth.
2. Include the nuts and dried natural product, mix and cover to stew just until the dried organic products have warmed. Sliced crisp organic product to add on top. Put in then sprinkle honey all.

7. Low Fat Tasty Cinnamon Nut Granola

Ingredients

- 2 mugs oats
- 2 mugs, puffed corn
- 2 mugs, puffed millet
- 1/2 cup cut almonds, walnuts or pistachios
- 3/4 cup dried cranberries or raisins
- 1/2 cup unsweetened fruit purée
- 1/4 cup honey/maple syrup
- 1 dropper loaded with Stevia fluid sweetener (discretionary)
- 2 tsp. cinnamon
- 1 tsp. vanilla
- salt
- 1/2 cup shredded coconut (discretionary)

Method:

1. Pre-heat broiler to 300 degrees
2. Measure oats, puffed corn and millet into a vast bowl and include nuts.
3. In a little bowl, include fruit purée, honey or maple syrup, cinnamon, vanilla and salt and blend well.
4. Add fluid Ingredients to the oats and mix to consolidate.
5. Spread on two heating sheets secured with material paper.
6. Heat for 30-45 minutes turning at regular intervals until delicately sautéed.

INSULIN RESISTANCE

7. Include dried organic product (and shredded coconut if utilizing) and mix.

8. Healthy Oat and Quinoa Cereal

Ingredients

- 2 mugs water
- 1/3 tsp cinnamon
- 1/3 tsp vanilla concentrate
- 1/4 tsp salt
- 1/2 glass moved oats
- 1/3 glass quinoa drops
- 1/3 glass plain yogurt
- 3 tsp honey
- 1/2 glass solidified berries, defrosted

Method

1. Add water to pan alongside the oats, quinoa, cinnamon, vanilla and salt.
2. Heat to the point of boiling, lower the warmth and cook until thickened.
3. Serve in a dish alongside half of the yogurt, half of the berries and a sprinkle of honey.
4. Appreciate

9. Sweet Healthy Potato Hash Browns

Ingredients

- 2 big sweet potatoes or yams, slashed
- 1 big onion, slashed
- 1 big red or green pepper, slashed
- 1/2 tsp. Smokey paprika (discretionary)
- 1/2 tsp. salt or to taste
- Pepper to taste

Method:

1. Preheat a big nonstick skillet and include the onions. Cook until they begin to cocoa somewhat.
2. Include the pepper, potatoes and flavors and keep on cooking, turning every now and again so as not to blaze. On the off chance that you have to, include a little water and cover to help the cooking procedure, yet reveal and let the water vanish before serving.
3. Salt and pepper to taste.

10. Healthy Pumpkin Chia Pudding

Ingredients

- 2 glasses unsweetened natural almond milk
- 1 glass natural pumpkin puree
- 2 Tbs. almond margarine
- 1 tsp. vanilla concentrate
- 1/4 glass maple syrup or honey (*see note beneath: to eliminate the sugar, utilize 1 tsp. of fluid Stevia)
- 2 tsp. pumpkin zest (or utilize 1 tsp cinnamon, 1/4 tsp ginger, squeeze ground clove, squeeze allspice
- 1/2 cup chia seeds found in most wellbeing sustenance stores.
- Discretionary Ingredients: pumpkin seeds, cleaved walnuts or pecans, shredded coconut or little chocolate chips.

Method:

1. Pour some almond milk into a glass bowl and include pumpkin puree. speed until the puree is totally broken down.
2. Include the almond spread, vanilla, maple syrup * and pumpkin zest and race till consolidated.
3. Include remaining almond drain and start including the chia seeds, speeding to blend.
4. Let stand for 5 minutes and after that rush to join the chia seeds all through the pudding.
5. Place in the fridge for 15 minutes then expel and whisk once more.

INSULIN RESISTANCE

6. Chill in the ice chest for around 30 minutes to permit the pudding to set.

11. Amazing Muesli

Ingredients

- 2 glasses oats
- 1 glass wheat pieces (Uncle Sam Brand)
- 1 glass quinoa Flakes (found close to the hot grains)
- 1/2 glass hemp hearts
- 1/2 glass ground flax seeds
- 1/2 glass fragmented almonds or entire almonds, cut
- 1/2 glass crude pumpkin seeds
- 1/2 glass walnuts
- 1/2 glass coconut pieces
- 1/2 glass raisins or other dried natural product (raisins have no sugar)
- 1 tsp. cinnamon
- 1 tsp. almond separate

Method

1. Put the majority of the Ingredients in a substantial bowl and mix to consolidate.
2. Store in a glass jug or compartment with a tight top.
3. Present with soy yogurt, berries and non-dairy milk.

INSULIN RESISTANCE

12. Chocolate Chip Tasty Pumpkin Muffins

Ingredients

- 1 medium banana, squashed
- 1 (15-oz.) can sweet pumpkin puree
- 1/4 glass 100% immaculate maple syrup
- 1 tsp. vanilla concentrate
- 2 mugs entire oat flour
- 1/2 tsp. heating pop
- 1/2 tsp. heating powder
- 1/2 tsp. salt
- 1 tsp. ground cinnamon
- 1/2 tsp. ground nutmeg
- 1/4 tsp. ground ginger
- 1 glass grain-sweetened sans dairy chocolate chips

Method

1. Preheat broiler to 375°F. In a big dish, join crushed banana, pumpkin puree, maple syrup, and vanilla concentrate.
2. In a little bowl, consolidate oat flour, preparing pop, heating powder, salt, cin-namon, nutmeg, and ginger. Exchange blend to extensive bowl and combine tenderly until very much joined. Maintain a strategic distance from over-blending to avert durability in the last item. Fold in chocolate chips.
3. Spoon player into silicon biscuit glasses and heat for 20 minutes or until the biscuits are gently cooked. Expel

biscuits from the broiler and let cool for 5 minutes. Store biscuits in a water/air proof holder.

INSULIN RESISTANCE

DRESSING RECIPES

13. HEALTHY VEGAN MUSHROOM GRAVY

INGREDIENTS

- 4 mugs low-sodium vegetable juices
- 1 cup slashed white onion
- 4 cloves garlic, finely cleaved
- 1 Tbl. tomato glue
- 8 ounces mushrooms, for example, porcini, cremini or shiitake, trimmed and slashed
- 2 Tbl. finely cleaved crisp thyme
- 1/2 finely cleaved crisp rosemary
- 1/3 cup red wine ideally something fiery like a Zen or Merlot
- 2 Tbl. diminished sodium tamari
- 2 Tbl. healthful yeast
- 2 Tbl. cornstarch
- Salt and pepper to taste

METHOD

1. Add onion to a huge skillet and sauté 3-4 minutes or until translucent. Include 1/4 measure of the stock to the skillet to keep onion from smoldering.

2. Include mushrooms and cook for 10-12 minutes or until they discharge their fluid and get to be delicate.
3. Mix in garlic, rosemary, thyme and tomato glue. Keep on cooking for 1 minute until fragrant.
4. Include wine and cook 1 minute, mixing always.
5. Mix in remaining 2 mugs juices and convey to a stew.
6. In a little bowl, whisk together tamari, nutritious yeast and cornstarch to shape a thick glue. Add blend to the skillet, whisking always to ensure glue breaks down. Heat blend to the point of boiling and cook 1 minute, mixing continually, until the sauce thickens.

14. Delicious Tahini Dressing

Ingredients

- 2 lemons
- 1 15-oz. can cannellini beans, washed
- 1/4 cup tahini
- 1/4 cup stone-ground mustard
- 3 Tbl. Braggs Amino Acids
- 2 Tbl. 100% unadulterated maple syrup
- 1/4 cup dietary yeast drops
- 1/2 cup water

Method:

1. Put all Ingredients into blender and mix until smooth.

15. Healthy Green Goddess Dressing

Ingredients

- 1/4 cup tahini
- 1/4 cup avocado
- 1/2 cup water
- 2 Tablespoons new parsley or cilantro, sliced
- 2 Tablespoons green onions, cleaved
- 1/2 teaspoon ocean salt
- 3 cloves garlic (or 1/2 tsp. garlic powder)
- 1 teaspoon Tamari (or soy sauce)
- 2 Tablespoons new lemon juice
- 2 Tablespoons apple juice vinegar

Method

1. Consolidate the majority of the Ingredients into a blender or nourishment processor and mix until smooth and rich.
2. Modify flavoring to taste and include more water, if vital, until coveted composition is accomplished.
3. Serve instantly, or store in the ice chest for up to 4 days in a fixed compartment. This dressing will thicken up when chilled, making a pleasant veggie plunge, as well!

INSULIN RESISTANCE

16. Healthy Mexican Salad with Lime Cilantro Dressing

Ingredients

- 2 1/2 glasses cleaved romaine lettuce
- 1 can (15.5 oz) dark beans, flushed
- 1 glass cleaved tomato or cherry tomatoes
- 1 glass cleaved peeled jicama
- 1 glass new corn portions, uncooked (or solidified or canned)
- 3/4 glass daintily cut radishes
- An entire ready avocado, diced
- 1 red ringer pepper, cleaved
- 4-5 corn tortillas

Dressing:

- 1/3 glass new lime juice
- 2 Tbl. honey
- 2 Tbl. finely slashed new cilantro
- 1 garlic clove, peeled and minced
- 1 tsp slashed jalapeño pepper (discretionary)

Method

1. Stack 2-3 corn tortillas on a slicing board and chop down the middle. At that point cut into around 1/3" strips. Place the strips on a microwavable plate. Sprinkle or shower with water or apple juice vinegar and daintily

salt. Microwave for around 2 minutes. Check for freshness, remembering that the tortilla strips will get crunchier as they cool. Include additional time in the event that they aren't sufficiently firm.
2. Prepare all the plate of mixed greens Ingredients with the exception of the avocado and tortilla strips in a substantial dish.
3. In isolated dish, blend dressing Ingredients.
4. Pour dressing over plate of mixed greens. Season with salt and pepper to taste and hurl.
5. Top individual servings with avocado and the firm tortilla strips.

DESSERT RECIPES

17. Tasty Baked Pears with Cardamom

INGREDIENTS

- 1/4 cup white wine
- 1/2 tsp. ground cardamom
- 1 tsp. vanilla
- 2-4 firm ready pears, divided and seeded
- 1/2 T. lemon juice
- 2 T. sugar

METHOD

1. Preheat broiler to 400 degrees F. Join wine, cardamom and vanilla in 8" square preparing dish.
2. Place pears cut-side up in heating dish and pour lemon juice over. Sprinkle with sugar.
3. Spread skillet with foil, place on the center rack in the over, and heat 30 minutes, or until delicate.
4. Evacuate thwart and move cup to top rack. Cook 5 less, or until delicately sautéed. Observe precisely.
5. Exchange pears to a serving place and sprinkle with juice from the dish.

18. Amazing Raspberry Jello

Ingredients

- 2 bundles solidified raspberries, defrosted.
- 1 some water
- 8 ounces (1 cup) vegetarian sharp cream or plain soy yogurt (6 oz)
- ½ cup walnuts
- 3 Tbl. Agar-agar chips (in the Asian area of the supermarket)
- ½ tsp. fluid stevia (orange seasoned)
- 1/8 cup maple syrup or other sugar

Method

1. Channel the fluid from the defrosted raspberries and place them in an extensive dish. Add the fluid to water to make 1 ½ glasses.
2. Heat water/raspberry juice in a little pot and include agar-agar. Mix until break down then put aside to cool for a couple of minutes.
3. Meanwhile, include the sharp cream or soy yogurt to the dish of raspberries alongside the walnuts.
4. At the point when the agar-agar has broken down. Add it to the dish of raspberries. Sir to join totally.
5. Refrigerate in this bowl, a mold or little serving holders until it is set.

INSULIN RESISTANCE

19. Healthy Strawberry Ice Cream

INGREDIENTS

- 3 bananas, peeled, unpleasant slashed, put into baggies and solidified
- 1 pack of solidified natural strawberries
- 2/3 glass crude cashews, doused for a few hours
- 4 set medjool dates (discretionary)
- 1 glass almond milk (or any milk elective you like)

METHOD

1. Put solidified bananas, strawberries, depleted and drenched cashews, dates, and almond milk into the cup of a powerful blender.
2. Mix, killing as often as possible to rub down the sides and help the blender to work.
3. Include more drain on the off chance that it appears to be too thick.
4. Serve quickly or fill a cooler safe dish and stop. You should give it a chance to defrost a little to recover the frozen yogurt to smoothness.
5. Top with walnuts or pistachios and cut strawberries, in the event that you like.

KATYA JOHANSSON

20. Chocolate Chip Tasty Chickpea Cookies

Ingredients

- 1, 15 oz can chickpeas, depleted
- 1/2 cup almond margarine (or nutty spread)
- 1/2 cup honey or maple syrup
- 1/3 cup oat flour
- 1 Tb. vanilla
- 1 tsp. cinnamon
- 2 tsp. preparing powder
- 1/2 tsp. salt
- 1/2 cup chocolate chips
- 1/2 cup slashed walnuts

Method

1. Preheat oven to 350 degrees and line a treat sheet with material paper.
2. Include chickpeas, almond spread, honey, flour, vanilla, cinnamon, heating powder and salt to the dish of a sustenance processor.
3. Process until blend is totally smooth, scratching down the sides to fuse all.
4. Expel to a dish and blend in chocolate chips and walnuts.
5. Drop by teaspoons onto material paper and spread them out somewhat with the back of your spoon.
6. Prepare for 25 minutes or until the sides turn somewhat cocoa. I like those crunchy bits and the inside of the treat with be chewy.

INSULIN RESISTANCE

21. Indian Spicy Carrot Pudding

Ingredients

- 5-6 peeled and shredded carrots
- 1/2 glasses unsweetened almond milk
- 1 glass light coconut milk
- 1/2 chia seeds
- 1/4 glass maple syrup or honey (to decrease the sugar, include 1/8 cup honey or syrup in addition to 1/3 tsp. fluid stevia)
- 1 tsp. vanilla concentrate
- 1/3 tsp. ground cardamom
- 1/4 tsp. ground ginger
- 1/2 tsp. ground cinnamon
- 1/4 tsp. ground cloves

Method

1. Place the shredded carrots and 1/2 cup almond in addition to 1/2 glass coconut milk in a pot over medium warmth. Include the flavors and cook until the carrots are delicate, around 20 minutes. Put aside to cool for a couple of minutes.
2. At the point when the carrots are somewhat cooled, include them and the cooking fluid to a blender and mix until smooth, including a portion of the almond milk to thin in the event that it gets too thick.
3. Include the rest of the milks and the sweetener and mix slower to consolidate.
4. Fill an extensive bowl and include the chia seeds, blending great.

5. Put the dish into the cooler to cool, stirring after around 15 minutes to ensure the chia seeds stay suspended. Keep on cooling until set.
6. Serve in individual bowls and top with cleaved walnuts, pumpkin seeds or scaled down chocolate chips.

22. Blueberry Lemon Tasty Coconut Bars

Ingredients

- 6 Tbl. new lemon juice
- 3 Tbl. chia seeds
- 1/2 cups antiquated oats, ground into flour in a blender
- 1/2 cup antiquated oats
- 2 Tbl. lemon get-up-and-go
- 1 cup shredded coconut
- 1 tsp. preparing powder
- 1/2 tsp salt
- 1/2 cup walnuts, sliced
- 1 cup solidified or new blueberries
- 2/3 cup fruit purée
- 1/4 cup coconut oil, dissolved
- 1/3 cup honey or maple syrup

Method

1. Heat the stove to 350 degrees and line a 8 x 8" preparing dish with material paper.
2. In a little bowl, blend the chia seeds with the lemon squeeze and put aside to thicken.
3. Blend the dry Ingredients, oat flour, oats, coconut, preparing powder, salt, with the walnuts and blueberries in an extensive dish.
4. Blend the wet Ingredients, the fruit purée, coconut oil, honey or maple syrup and absorbed chia seeds another dish.

5. Empty the dry Ingredients into the wet and blend until consolidated. You may utilize your hands to ensure all is joined. The batter will be really dry.
6. Press the mixture into your readied dish, leveling the top with your spoon.
7. Heat in your preheated broiler for around 30 minutes or until the edges start to cocoa.
8. Let cool before expelling from the skillet. Cut into squares.

INSULIN RESISTANCE

23. HEALTH BLACK BEAN BROWNIES

INGREDIENTS

- 15 ounces no-salt dark beans, depleted and washed
- 2 ready medium estimated bananas
- 1/4 cup maple syrup
- 1/4 cup sugar
- 1/4 cup unsweetened cacao. I incline toward the KIVA brand.
- 1/2 Tbl. cinnamon
- 1 tsp. vanilla concentrate
- 1/2 glass customary or non-dairy chocolate chips
- 1/2 glass cleaved walnuts (discretionary)
- 1/2 glass moment oats or oat flour (made in a sustenance processor from crude oats)

METHOD

1. Preheat broiler to 350 degrees F. Gently coat a 8×6? Sprinkle with cooking spray.
2. Join all Ingredients, aside from oats, chocolate chips and walnuts in a nourishment processor. Mix until smooth.
3. Mix in the oat flour/oats until mixed well. Fold in chocolate chips and nuts. Empty player into the cup. Prepare 30-35 minutes or until a toothpick confesses all.

LUNCH RECIPES

24. Gluten-Free Tasty Sandwich Bread

INGREDIENTS

- 1/2 cups millet flour
- 1/2 cups oat flour (ensure you purchase one that is named sans gluten)
- 1/2 cup rice flour
- 1/2 cup tapioca starch
- 1/4 cup flax dinner
- 2 tbsp egg replacer (can substitute corn starch)
- 2 tbsp xanthan gum
- 1/2 tsp preparing pop
- 1/4 cups warm water
- 2 1/4 tsp of dynamic dry yeast (1 bundle)
- 1 cup almond milk blended with 1 tsp vinegar
- 1 tbsp maple syrup (can substitute sugar)
- 1/2 tsp finely ground ocean salt
- 2 tbsp olive oil

METHOD:

1. Include the yeast and maple syrup to the water and let stand until the yeast begins to sprout, around 5-10 minutes.

INSULIN RESISTANCE

2. Combine the different flours with the heating pop, flax dinner, egg replacer, and xanthan gum. Whisk everything altogether to guarantee it's all combined.
3. Add the almond milk to the yeast-water blend alongside the flours and salt.
4. Blend utilizing the oar connection on a stand blender or by hand. Sprinkle in the oil as you blend. Keep on mixing for around 8 minutes or until everything's all around consolidated and you have a genuinely smooth-looking, player like mixture.
5. Oil a standard 9 by 5 inch piece dish. Empty the batter into the cup and, utilizing a spatula, even out the top as well as can be expected.
6. Spread with a kitchen towel and let it ascend in a warm place for 60-a hour and a half or until the mixture has domed around the highest point of the dish.
7. Preheat the stove to 350 degrees Fahrenheit and prepare the bread for 55 minutes. Embed a thermometer in the center toward the end of baking– it ought to enlist no less than 200 degrees.
8. Expel the chunk from the stove and let it stand on a rack until sufficiently cool to handle, around 20 minutes. Expel from the roll skillet and keep cooling the bread on the rack.

25. ROASTED TASTY BUDDHA BOWL

INGREDIENTS

- 1 broccoli, cut into florets
- 1 cauliflower, cut into florets
- extensive modest bunch radishes, split (or quartered relying upon the size)
- 1 – 2 tablespoons olive oil or sesame oil
- liberal sprinkle of garlic powder
- squeeze or two of salt
- Smooth Lemon White Bean Sauce
- 1 can (15 oz) cannellini beans, depleted and washed
- 2 tablespoons tahini
- 2 tablespoons additional virgin olive oil
- 2 tablespoons nutritious yeast, discretionary
- 1 huge garlic clove
- juice of 1 huge lemon
- salt to taste
- 2 – 4 tablespoons water for diminishing

METHOD

1. Preheat stove to 400 degrees.
2. In a huge dish, consolidate broccoli, cauliflower and radishes, sprinkle with oil, garlic powder and salt, blend well to coat. Place blend on rimmed treat sheet or broiling dish. Cook for 30-40 minutes, mixing once in the middle.
3. Set you up sauce by setting every one of the Ingredients in nourishment processor/blender, aside from the water, and mix until rich smooth. Include water 1 tablespoon at

INSULIN RESISTANCE

once until wanted consistency. You may likewise jump at the chance to include more lemon set up of water for a truly fiery lemon sauce. Taste for flavor including additional garlic or salt if necessary.
4. Serve vegetables on top of grain of decision (I utilized quinoa) and include a liberal measure of sauce on top. Include some naturally split pepper in the event that you like.

26. Tasty Vegetable Fritters

Ingredients

- 1/2 cup flour
- 1/2 cup soy milk, or other without dairy milk
- 1 corn cob, cut the corn parts off the cob
- 1/2 big zucchini, ground
- 1/2 carrot, ground
- 2 broccoli florets, finely slashed
- 1 spring onion, finely cut
- Salt and pepper

Method

1. Blend the flour and soy milk to shape a player.
2. Blend through the veggies and season well with salt and pepper.
3. Heat an big griddle over a high warmth and include a little oil. Include a tablespoon of the blend to the dish at once, forming into little adjusts. Cook the wastes until cocoa on one side then flip over deliberately and cook the other side.
4. Channel on kitchen paper and serve instantly.

27. Healthy Bean and Vegetable Chili

Ingredients

- 1 medium onion — coarsely sliced
- 1 green chime pepper — cored, seeded and diced
- 2 cloves garlic — minced
- 3 cups pinto beans*, cooked — (or 2 jars)
- 2 14.5 ounce jars diced tomatoes — (I utilized 1 can w/green chilies, 1 can normal)
- 2 teaspoons stew powder
- 1 teaspoon cumin
- 1/2 cups corn — crisp or solidified
- 1/4 teaspoon salt — (discretionary, to taste)
- 1/2 cups zucchini — diced (around 2 medium)

Method

1. In a non-stick dish over medium warmth, sauté the onion, ringer pepper and garlic just until softly cooked, around 3 minutes.
2. Include the beans, tomatoes, and seasonings. Heat to the point of boiling, then lessen warmth, and stew revealed for around 10 minutes. Mix in the corn and zucchini and keep on cooking until the zucchini is only delicate, not soft, around 7 minutes.

KATYA JOHANSSON

28. Tasty Jackfruit Chicken Noodle Soup

Ingredients

- 1 jar of jackfruit in salt water
- 1 medium carrot
- 1 stalk of celery
- 1 little onion
- 1 clove of garlic
- 2 bouillon shapes
- 1 glass dry noodles
- some water

Method

1. Shredding the Jackfruit to make the "chicken" you'll need to open and deplete the jar of jackfruit and add that to a dish. Include some bubbling water and one bouillon 3D shape. Give that a chance to sit for 60 minutes or thereabouts. The thought here is that the jackfruit absorb some of that flavor. Once you've given it a chance to sit for some time, then start up the stove. In a skillet, include two or three tablespoons of oil. We utilize sunflower or safflower oil in light of the fact that their flavors are mellow and won't meddle with our flavoring. Precisely include the jackfruit and sear until every side tans. Save that juices. Once the jackfruit tans you'll need to take a few forks to shred it.
2. Jackfruit stewing in stock once it is all shredded then add the other bouillon solid shape to the spared measure

INSULIN RESISTANCE

of soup. Add this to the skillet and stew until the vast majority of the fluid is cooked off. Now your "chicken" is prepared for the soup. You can broil it in your stove to toughen up the surface more if sought.
3. Jackfruit For whatever remains of the soup you just need to make some Mirepoix, include the "chicken" and more juices, and whatever noodles you lean toward.

29. Bean Sald

Ingredients

- 2 tablespoons balsamic vinegar
- 2 tablespoons tomato ketchup
- 3 teaspoons maple syrup
- 3 garlic cloves (pulverized then finely slashed)
- 1 red onion (finely cleaved)
- 425g/15oz can red kidney beans (depleted and washed)
- 425g/15oz can cannellini beans (depleted and washed)
- 4 tablespoons new level lead parsley (finely slashed)

Method

1. Put the balsamic vinegar, tomato ketchup, maple syrup, garlic and 2 tablespoons of water into a dish and blend.
2. Include the onion and beans and blend into the dressing until every one of the beans all covered. Include a little Maldon ocean salt and dark pepper to taste and chill.
3. Just before serving include the crisp parsley.

30. Tasty Tabbouleh

Ingredients

- 225g/8oz bulgur wheat
- gigantic group of crisp parsley (stalks evacuated, washed, flushed and finely slashed)
- 10 sprigs of crisp mint (stalks expelled, washed, flushed and finely slashed)
- 4 spring onions/scallions (trimmed and finely sliced)
- juice of one lemon
- Maldon ocean salt
- naturally ground dark pepper

Method

1. Take after the cooking guidelines for the bulgur wheat on the bundle. This generally implies putting the bulgur wheat in a dish and covering it with bubbling water and giving it a chance to sit for around 20 - 30 minutes.
2. Once the wheat is prepared and you've arranged alternate Ingredients, quite recently include the parsley, mint, spring onion and lemon juice to the wheat and combine. Include somewhat more lemon juice in the event that you need. Season with salt and pepper then cover and chill until you're prepared to utilize it.

KATYA JOHANSSON

31. Delicious Red Pepper, Chickpea and Spinach Soup

Ingredients

- 1 onion (finely slashed)
- 2 garlic cloves, squashed
- 1 red pepper (finely slashed)
- 1 teaspoon cumin seeds
- 375ml/1.5 glasses tomato passata
- 750ml/3 glasses Marigold Vegan Bouillon
- 300g/10.5oz chickpeas (flushed and depleted in case you're utilizing the canned assortment)
- 2 teaspoons red wine vinegar
- 100g/3.5oz spinach leaves (washed)
- naturally ground dark pepper

Method

1. Cook the onion and garlic in 2cm or 1 inch of water for five minutes until delicate. On the off chance that the water dissipates too rapidly, simply include somewhat more.
2. Include the red pepper and cumin seeds. Blend and cook for a further 2 minutes.
3. Include the passata and stock, convey to the come then turn down and stew for 10 minutes.
4. Include the chickpeas, vinegar and cook for a further five minutes.

INSULIN RESISTANCE

5. Add the spinach and season to taste with naturally ground dark pepper. Cook until the spinach starts to shrivel, then serve into warm soup bowls.

32. Spicy Tasty Hummus

Ingredients

- 4 garlic cloves
- 2 cups canned chickpeas, drained, liquid reserved
- 1 1/2 teaspoons kosher salt
- 1/3 cup tahini (sesame paste)
- 6 tablespoons freshly squeezed lemon juice (2 lemons)
- 2 tablespoons water or liquid from the chickpeas
- hot sauce

Method

1. Turn on the food processor fitted with the steel blade and drop the garlic down the feed tube; process until it's minced.
2. Add the rest of the ingredients to the food processor and process until the hummus is coarsely pureed. Taste, for seasoning, and serve chilled or at room temperature.

INSULIN RESISTANCE

33. Healthy Chickpea, Lentil and Spinach Stew

Ingredients

- 1 Large Onion (Finely Chopped)
- 3 Garlic Cloves (Crushed)
- 3cm Fresh Ginger (Finley Grated)
- 3 teaspoons Ground Coriander
- 2 teaspoons Ground Cumin
- 1/2 teaspoon Chili Powder (Choose your most loved quality)
- 1 tin Chopped Tomatoes
- 850ml Marigold Vegan Bouillion
- 250g Red Lentils (Washed until the water runs clear)
- 1 tin Chickpeas in water (Drained)
- 250g Fresh Spinach (Finely cut into 1cm strips)
- 250g Fresh kale (Finely cut into 1cm strips)
- 1 glass Brown Rice (Per Person)

Method

1. Put the slashed onions in a cup with around 3cm of water and mellow over a low eat for 5-7 minutes then include the pulverized garlic and cook tenderly for one more moment.
2. Include every one of the flavors and cook for a further moment. On the off chance that it looks as if it will get on add a little water to free it up.
3. Include the lentils, tomatoes, stock and stew revealed for around 20 minutes. Check to guarantee the lentils are

cooked, on the off chance that they're still somewhat hard cook for a further 5 minutes. Include more stock in the event that you have to.
4. Flush the brown rice and cook in bubbling water according to the bundle Method, for the most part for around 20-25 minutes.
5. Include the chickpeas and cook for a further 7 minutes then include the kale for a further two minutes lastly the spinach for two more minutes.
6. Channel the brown rice and invigorate under bubbling water until the water runs clear. Plate up the chickpea and spinach stew with the brown rice.
7. Press a little lemon juice over the stew for included punch. Appreciate!

34. Amazing Spicy Bean Spread

Ingredients

- 400g/14oz blended beans e.g. kidney, dark, haricot (If you're utilizing a can, deplete and wash them)
- 1 tablespoon tomato puree
- Worcestershire sauce (no fish form) to taste
- Tabasco to taste
- One teaspoon smashed dried chilies
- Half teaspoon ground cumin
- Half teaspoon ground coriander
- 2 tablespoons new rosemary, cleaved
- 6 child tomatoes, cleaved

Method

1. Put every one of the Ingredients aside from the rosemary and infant tomatoes into a dish and pound either with a fork, or I utilized a hand blender.
2. Include the child tomatoes and the crisp, slashed rosemary and blend in.
3. Use as a spread on whatever you pick - toast, flatbread, ciabatta, inside a pitta or as a filling for a prepared potato. Present with a green plate of mixed greens for a yummy filling lunch.

DINNER RECIPES

35. Healthy Crispy Cauliflower

INGREDIENTS

- 1 head cauliflower, cut into florets, stem cut into little pieces
- 2 Tbsp potato starch
- 1/2 tsp salt
- 1/4 tsp dark pepper
- 1/2 tsp turmeric
- 1 Tbsp healthful yeast, discretionary
- 1/2 tsp bean stew powder or paprika
- 1 Tbsp nonpartisan, high warmth oil of decision (avocado, sunflower, grape seed, canola, and so on)

METHOD

1. Preheat broiler to 450 degrees. Sprinkle tablespoon of oil over metal preparing sheet. Spread cauliflower over sheet, hurl in oil, and sprinkle with remaining Ingredients, potato starch through bean stew powder/paprika. Ensure cauliflower is in an even layer with however much space between pieces as could reasonably be expected. If necessary partition between two sheets.
2. Heat for 20-30 minutes, hurling once about part of the way through. Whenever firm and brilliant cocoa it is finished. Serve without anyone else's input, over rice,

INSULIN RESISTANCE

pasta, with potatoes, or as a filling for tacos, burritos, wraps, and so forth. Shower with balsamic vinegar, tahini dressing, or aioli if fancied. Appreciate!

KATYA JOHANSSON

36. Healthy Potato Lentil Turmeric Soup

Ingredients

- 2 glasses potatoes, unpeeled and cubed (reddish brown or yukon gold)
- 1 medium yellow onion, diced
- 2 cloves garlic, slashed
- 1" bit of ginger, peeled and slashed
- 1 glass red lentils
- 4 glasses vegetable stock (around 1 cup)
- 1 Tbsp cumin seed, entirety
- 1 Tbsp cocoa mustard seeds
- 1 tsp salt, or more to taste
- 1 Tbsp medium-high warmth oil
- 1/2 tsp turmeric
- 1/2 tsp dark pepper
- squeeze cayenne pepper if wanted
- discretionary: 1 cup canned coconut milk, for included smoothness

Method

1. In a huge soup pot, or dutch stove, heat oil over medium warmth. Include mustard seeds and cumin seeds. Heat until mustard seeds start to pop, around 1-2 minutes. Try not to let cumin seeds smolder.
2. Include onion, garlic, and ginger. Cook over medium-low warmth with cover on for 2-3 minutes until onion starts to mollify. Include potatoes and red lentils and mix to

INSULIN RESISTANCE

     coat. Add stock and convey to a delicate stew. Spread pot and cook over medium low warmth for 15-20 minutes until potatoes and lentils are delicate and mashable.
3. Include salt, dark pepper and turmeric to taste. In the event that utilizing coconut milk mix as a part of to fuse now. The soup will be stout now. Eat as seems to be, or utilize a drenching blender to mix until rich. You can likewise utilize a general blender, however you will need to mix in clumps once the soup has cooled a bit. Keep warm on low warmth. Solidifies well!

37. Five Minute Fresh Tasty Salsa

Ingredients

- 1 glass ready cherry tomatoes, or 2-3 ready plum tomatoes, coarsely slashed
- 2 Tbsp white or red onion, or shallot, coarsely slashed
- 1 medium clove crisp garlic, peeled and coarsely slashed
- 1 little jalapeño, coarsely slashed, seeds evacuated in the event that you incline toward mellow salsa
- 1 Tbsp olive oil, discretionary
- 1/4 glass crisp cilantro, coarsely sliced
- juice from a large portion of a lime, or to taste
- squeeze of salt, to taste
- Discretionary increases: poblano, chipotle, or red ringer pepper, pineapple or mango

Method

1. Put all Ingredients tomatoes through olive oil (if utilizing), into a blender or nourishment processor and mix until rich, or leave all the more coarsely cleaved in the event that you lean toward.
2. Include cilantro and process again for a brief moment or two to convey equally. Season with lime squeeze and salt to taste and chill or serve instantly.

38. Tasty Baked Sesame Fries

Ingredients

- 1 lb. Yukon gold potatoes, unpeeled, cut into wedges
- 1 Tbsp medium-high warmth oil, avocado, grape seed, sunflower, and so forth.
- 2 Tbsp sesame seeds
- 1 Tbsp potato starch, discretionary, however makes fries additional firm
- 1 Tbsp wholesome yeast, discretionary
- liberal squeeze of salt, to taste
- dark pepper to taste

Method

1. Preheat broiler to 425 degrees. Delicately oil metal heating sheet, or cover with material paper. Hurl potatoes in all Ingredients until covered, if seeds don't stick, shower with more oil.
2. Spread potatoes on preparing sheet in an even layer (the more space between the wedges the better) and heat for 20-25 minutes, flipping once part of the way through, until potatoes are brilliant cocoa and firm. Serve quickly with toppings of decision. Appreciate!

39. Healthy Chickpeas and Rice

Ingredients

- 1 cup grain rice (or cocoa rice)
- 1 can chickpeas, depleted and washed
- 4-5 child Portobello mushrooms, diced
- 1/2 cup vegetarian grill sauce - I utilized my formula from this post
- sriracha or other hot sauce (discretionary)
- cilantro or parsley, to embellish

Method

1. Cook brown rice as indicated by the bundle Method. I get a kick out of the chance to utilize a rice cooker for this reason.
2. Preheat the stove to 375 degrees.
3. Add chickpeas and mushrooms to an ovenproof dish (Pyrex dishes are my go to). Pour grill sauce over the blend, mix, and send to the preheated stove.
4. Prepare for 15-20 min, mixing several times, until the sauce dissipates marginally however doesn't dry out totally. Take the chickpeas out of the broiler, blend in hot sauce (if utilizing), and let rest for 5 min.
5. To serve: Arrange cooked rice on a plate, top with chickpeas, trim with cilantro or parsley.

40. Tasty Peanut Butter from Scratch

Ingredients

- 1 lb. crude peeled peanuts
- 1-2 Tbsp ground flaxseed
- Squeeze of salt, to taste
- Discretionary:
- Other crude or broiled unsalted nuts (walnuts, almonds, and so forth.)
- Honey

Method

To set up the peanuts:
1. Preheat the stove to 350°F. Spread peanuts in a solitary layer on a foil-lined treat sheet/pizza skillet. Broil for 14-16 min, contingent upon how hot your stove gets. Shake the dish enthusiastically halfway through simmering.
2. When peanuts are done, permit to cool for no less than 1-2 hours. At the point when sufficiently cool to handle, peel off the red skins by rubbing a modest bunch at once between the palms of your hands. Put peeled peanuts in a different dish, or straight into the dish of your nourishment processor/blender.

To make smooth nutty spread:
3. Include peeled peanuts and whatever remains of the Ingredients to the nourishment processor/blender. Mix

for 5-6 min, scratching off the sides frequently, until the nutty spread is smooth. Just before it's done, taste and change the saltiness/sweetness to your preferring.
4. Store in a lidded holder in the refrigerator. Stays useful for 1-2 weeks or more (see note).
5. To make crunchy nutty spread:
6. Take after the progressions for smooth nutty spread, however spare a modest bunch of peeled peanuts when putting whatever is left of them in your sustenance processor. Just before your nutty spread is done, include the spared peanuts and heartbeat the processor 2-3 times, or until the lumps are the right size to your taste. Store the same way.

41. Amazing Creamy Mushroom Pasta

Ingredients

- 2 cups of Sliced Mushrooms
- 2 cups of Broccoli chopped into large thumb sized pieces
- 125 gr pf Pasta uncooked, any type you like
- 1/4 tsp. of celtic sea salt optional, to taste
- 1/4 tsp. of Pepper or to taste
- 2 tsp. of Dried Herbs / chives
- 3 tsp. of Nutritional Yeast Flakes optional, but adds nice cheesy flavor
- 2 tsp. of Tahini Paste
- 3 tsp. of Brown Rice Flour or Corn Starch
- 500 ml of Plant Milk any unsweetened plant based milk that you like
- 500 ml of Water or Vegetable Broth or Extra Plant Milk

Method

1. Get a medium sized pot with a lid and place in all of the ingredients prior to putting on the heat.
2. Give everything a good mix through and turn the heat on to a medium-high heat and stir through occasionally until it reaches a light boil.
3. Once it reaches a light boil, place the lid on the pot and keep it at low boil for about 5 minutes.
4. Remove the lid and stir. Add extra water, stir again and let it continue to cook with a lid on until your pasta is

cooked through. Check your packet Method as to how long it will need. (Usually between 8 to 12 minutes).

42. Delicious Vegan Pizza

Ingredients

- 2 tbsp Whole wheat Flour or flour of choice
- 1/8 tsp Baking Powder
- 1 pinch coarse celtic sea salt
- 2 tbsp Filtered Water
- Toppings
- 1 tsp Tomato Paste or Thick Pasta Sauce
- 1-2 tbsp Chopped tomato
- 3 whole Pimento Stuffed Olives, sliced
- 1 large Button Mushroom, sliced
- Any herbs and spices or toppings of your choice OPTIONAL
- "Cheesy" Topping
- 2 tsp Filtered Water
- 2 tsp Nutritional Yeast Flakes
- 1 tsp White Miso paste
- 2 tsp Tahini (sesame paste)

Method

1. Place all of the pizza base ingredients into a mug or large cup and stir until all the ingredients are mixed well and resemble a batter. This will take about half a minute to a minute.
2. Plop the tomato paste over the top and then place the other toppings evenly over the top also.
3. Add all of the Cheesy Topping ingredients in a small bowl and stir until smooth and mixed together. Pour this evenly over your pizza toppings.

4. Place in the microwave for 1 minute and check if the base has cooked. If it needs a bit longer, place it back in 10 seconds at a time until done. Enjoy!

43. Tasty Alfredo Potato Bake

Bake Ingredients
- 7 large Boiled Potatoes, peeled and cooled sliced thinly
- 1 medium to large White Onion sliced thinly
- Nutmeg or Parika to sprinkle over the top

Alfredo Sauce Ingredients
- 1 1/2 cups Filtered Water
- 1/2 cups Plant Milk (I used organic soy milk) or unsweetened plant milk of choice
- 1 large Boiled Potato, peeled
- 1 tbsp Miso paste (soy, chickpea or brown rice miso)
- 1/2 cups Nutritional Yeast Flakes
- 1 tsp Garlic Powder
- 1 tsp Onion Powder
- 1/2 tsp coarse Celtic sea salt optional, to taste only
- 1/4 tsp White Pepper
- 1 tbsp Tahini
- 750 g Steamed Cauliflower (1 medium head)

Method

1. Preheat oven to 200C/400F.
2. Layer potato and onion in a 2 Qt/2 Liter size casserole dish (with lid). Finish with a layer of potato.
3. Next, place all of the Alfredo sauce ingredients into a blender. Blend on high for a minute or two until smooth and creamy.
4. Pour the Alfredo sauce evenly over the potatoes, making sure that the sauce runs down and around the sides of the potatoes. Lightly sprinkle with nutmeg or paprika,

and cover with a lid. If you do not have a baking dish with a lid, use some aluminum foil to cover it tightly.
5. Bake in oven for 15 minutes. Remove the lid and place back in the oven for another 15 to 20 minutes until the potatoes are cooked through and the top is browned to your liking.

44. Healthy Black Bean with Potato Seitan Roast

Ingredients

- 3 slices Whole-wheat Bread Toasted and cut into thumb size pieces
- 2 whole Boiled Potatoes Skin removed and chopped into small pieces
- 400 grams Black Beans Cooked and drained. Canned is fine
- 1/4 cup Nutrional Yeast Flakes
- 1/4 cup Scallions Finely chopped
- 2 tbsp Dried Mixed Italian Herbs
- 1 tsp Garlic Powder
- 1 tbsp Granulated Onion
- 1/8 tsp Black Pepper (freshly ground)
- 2 cups Vegetable Stock Salted
- 1 tbsp Tamari or Soy Sauce
- 2 cups Gluten Flour - Vital Wheat Gluten

Method

1. For this recipe you will need a large mixing bowl, a potato masher (if you do not like mixing by hand), a large bread pan, non-stick parchment paper, aluminum foil and a baking tray.
2. Firstly, set your oven to 180 degrees C (360 F). Next take your large mixing bowl and add the toast, potatoes and black beans before mashing by hand or with masher.

3. Now add the flakes, scallions, dried herbs, garlic powder, granulated onion and pepper before mixing again. Now add the rest of the ingredients in order before kneading the roast until well combined (about 2 minutes). The mixture should be like a stringy dough. Depending on the moisture content of your potatoes, beans etc you may need more flour or water to get the mixture to the right consistency.
4. Line your bread pan with baking paper then fill with the mixture. Cover the pan with Aluminum foil and place in the oven for 30 minutes. After 30 minutes remove the foil and place back in the oven for a further 30 minutes.
5. After the hour is complete you should be able to remove the roast from the baking pan in one piece. My roast was still soft on the sides so I wrapped it in fresh baking paper and foil, placed it on a baking tray and cooked it for a further hour flipping the roast at the 30 minute mark.

INSULIN RESISTANCE

45. Vegan Cheesy Sweet Potato & Kale Bake

Bake Ingredients

- 600 g Sweet Potatoes sliced thinly
- 110 g Kale Leaves (or spinach if preferred) chopped small
- Paprika or nutmeg to sprinkle over the top
- Cheesy Sauce Ingredients
- 1/2 cups Almonds, blanched (or other nuts of choice) soaked for 30 mins in boiled hot water, then drained
- 2 cups Vegetable Stock
- 1/2 cups Plant Milk (I used organic soy milk) or unsweetened plant milk of choice
- 1 tbsp Miso paste (soy, chickpea or brown rice miso)
- 1 tsp Garlic Powder
- 1 tsp Granulated Onion (or onion flakes)
- 1/4 tsp White Pepper
- 1 tbsp Tahini
- coarse Celtic sea salt optional, to taste only

Method

1. Preheat oven to 200C/400F.
2. Place sweet potato and kale into a 2 Qt/2 Litre size casserole dish (with lid).
3. Next, place all of the cheesy sauce ingredients into a blender. Blend on high for a minute or two until smooth and creamy.
4. Pour the cheesy sauce evenly over the vegetables, lightly sprinkle with paprika or nutmeg. And cover with a lid. If

you do not have a baking dish with a lid, use some aluminum foil to cover it tightly.
5. Bake in oven for 30 minutes. Check the sweet potato to check how well it is cooked through. Place back in the oven for 10 to 20 minutes until the sweet potatoes are cooked through to your liking.

46. Healthy Chickpea with Potato Burger Patties

Ingredients

- 400 g Can Chickpeas, drained
- 600 g Boiled Potatoes, peeled and cooled approx. 3 to 4 large potatoes
- 400 g Eggplant, peeled and diced 1 small eggplant
- 60 g Onion, peeled and diced 1 small onion
- 1 small Handful Fresh Basil leaves or 1 tablespoon dried herbs of choice
- 1 tbsp Dried Onion Flakes
- 1 tsp coarse Celtic sea salt
- 1/4 - 1/2 tsp White Pepper
- Optional Add In - Only use this if you want slightly firmer burger patties!
- 1/4 cups Chickpea or Tapioca flour

Method

1. Stir fry the eggplant and onion using a few teaspoons of water or vegetable broth to stop them from sticking. Set aside once cooked through. NOTE: you could also bake in the oven until soft if you prefer.
2. Preheat oven to 180C/360F.
3. Next, place all of the ingredients into a food processor.
4. Pulse 3 times and then let it run for about 25 seconds.
5. Turn the food processor off and remove the blade from the machine.

6. Shape the mixture into 12 burger patties and place onto a large baking tray lined with non-stick parchment paper.
7. Bake in oven for 30 minutes. Turn, and bake again for a further 10 minutes or until you reach your desired level of brownness. Enjoy!

47. Amazing Pea and Mushroom Risotto

Ingredients

- 1 1/2 tbsp Cornstarch
- 1 cup Plant Milk (I used organic soy milk)
- 1 small Onion sliced
- 3 large Portobello Mushrooms sliced thickly
- 1 cup Frozen Peas
- 1 tbsp Dried Mixed Italian Herbs
- 1/2 tsp coarse Celtic sea salt
- 1/2 tsp Vegetable stock powder
- 1 cup Cooked Rice (mine was leftover from dinner the night before)
- Black Pepper to taste

Method

1. Put a non-stick fry pan on medium-high heat.
2. Mix the cornstarch and plant milk together in a screw top jar or in a mixing bowl until well combined. (See video at the top of this recipe for full demonstration). Set aside.
3. Add sliced onion into the heated pan. Stir until golden. Use a teaspoon of water if it sticks too much.
4. Add the sliced mushrooms and stir through. Add the peas and stir through again.
5. Add the herbs, sea salt and stock powder and continue to stir through to combine all of the flavors and ingredients thoroughly.

6. Add in the rice and stir through to heat it. Turn heat down to low-medium, then add the cornstarch/plant milk mixture to the pan. Stir until well combined and mixed together.
7. Turn heat off and let it sit on the residual heat for 5 minutes before serving.
8. Grind some fresh black pepper over the top to taste.

48. Amazing Seitan Roast

INGREDIENTS

- 480 grams Cooked Beans
- 100 grams Cooked Rice (or Quinoa)
- 3 tbs Tomato Paste
- 2 tsp Smoked Paprika
- 1 tsp Vegetable stock powder
- 2 tbs Tamari
- 1 tbs Dried Onion Flakes
- 1 tbs Dried Sage Leaves
- 80 grams Brown Rice Flour (1/2 metric cup)
- 40 grams chickpea flour/Besan Flour (1/4 metric cup)
- Black Pepper to taste

METHOD

1. Place the beans and cooked rice in a food processor and blend until reasonably smooth but still with some chunky texture.
2. Place bean and rice mixture in a mixing bowl and add all of the remaining ingredients. Mix well with your hands until it all holds together.
3. Preheat your oven to 180C/360F.
4. Place your mixture on some non-stick parchment paper and fold closed. Wrap in some aluminum foil and bake in oven for 45 minutes.

49. Roasted Garden Vegetables

Ingredients

- 1 bunch Baby Carrots
- 2 handfuls Green Beans top and tailed
- 1 large Onion cut into 8 wedges
- 15 fresh Cherry Tomatoes halved
- 3 sprigs Thyme
- 1 tsp Dried Onion Flakes
- 1 tsp Dried Sage Leaves
- 1/2 tsp coarse Celtic sea salt or to taste
- 1/8 tsp Black Pepper, ground or to taste
- 1/4 tsp chili flakes optional, to taste
- 200 ml Vegetable Broth
- 1 tbsp Tamari or soy sauce/Braggs Aminos

Method

1. Preheat oven to 175 degrees Celsius (350 degrees Fahrenheit).
2. Add vegetables to a roasting or baking pan. I used an 8 x 8 inch (20 x 20cm) glass dish.
3. Add spices and liquids to the dish.
4. Give a little stir through and place in oven.
5. Check every 15 to 20 minutes and give a stir through. Cook until vegetables are roasted to your liking. Mine took 1 hour.

50. Curried Delicious Rice Noodles

Ingredients

- 1 medium Red Bell Pepper (Capsicum) thinly sliced
- 1/4 cup Scallions thinly sliced
- 1 - 2 cloves Garlic chopped
- 1/4 cup Frozen Peas
- 1 tsp Tomato Paste
- 2 tsp Curry Powder
- 1/8 tsp Turmeric
- 1/8 tsp White Pepper
- 120 grams Rice Vermicelli Noodles cooked and drained
- 1/2 cup Vegetable Broth
- Salt and Chili optional, to taste

Method

1. Heat a non-stick fry pan to medium-high heat. Add peppers and stir until softened.
2. Add scallions and stir through again.
3. Add garlic and stir through for a minute or so. Then add the frozen peas and stir through for a minute more.
4. Add tomato paste and spices and continue to stir for another minute.
5. Toss through the noodles and add the vegetable broth to loosen everything from the pan and stir through until everything is well combined.

KATYA JOHANSSON

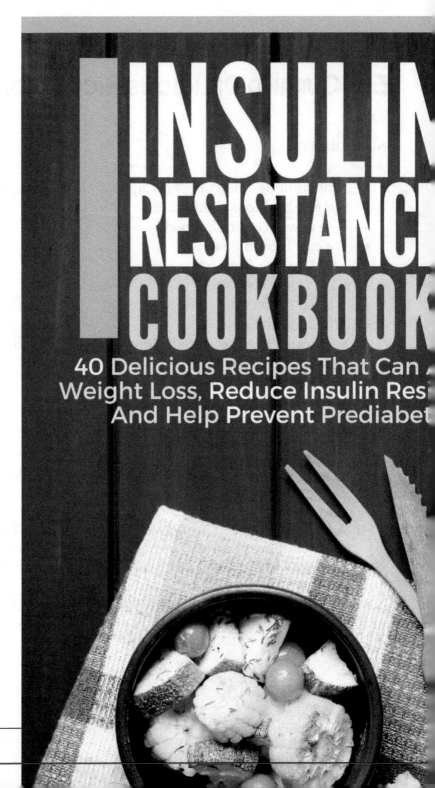

INSULIN RESISTANCE COOKBOOK

40 Delicious Recipes That Can Aid In Weight Loss, Reduce Insulin Resistance And Help Prevent Prediabetes

by
KATYA JOHANSSON

Copyright © 2016 by Katya Johansson.
All Rights Reserved.

More Books at www.katyajohansson.com

KATYA JOHANSSON

INSULIN RESISTANCE

INTRODUCTION

Insulin is a hormone made in the pancreas, an organ located behind the stomach. Its main role is to regulate the amount of nutrients circulating in the bloodstream.
Although insulin is mostly implicated in blood sugar management, it also affects fat and protein metabolism.

Sometimes our cells stop responding to insulin like they are supposed to. In other words, they become "resistant" to the insulin.
This condition is termed insulin resistance, and is very common.

Wikipedia's definition of insulin resistance is: "Insulin resistance (IR) is generally regarded as a pathological condition in which cells fail to respond to the normal actions of the hormone insulin. The body produces insulin when glucose starts to be released into the bloodstream from the digestion of carbohydrates in the diet. Normally this insulin response triggers glucose being taken into body cells, to be used for energy, and inhibits the body from using fat as energy".

When blood sugar levels exceed a certain threshold, a diagnosis of type 2 diabetes is made. In fact, this is a simplified version of how type 2 diabetes develops. Insulin resistance is the principal cause of this common disease.

The recommended diet for this condition is: green vegetables like broccoli, zucchini, eggplant, carrots, capsicum, celery, cucumber, lettuce, tomato, onion, shallot, leeks, green beans, asparagus, bok choy, choy sum, snow peas, mushrooms, bean sprouts, alfalfa sprouts, rhubarb, leeks, chives and if you can stomach them, you can have cauliflower, Brussel sprouts and cabbage.

KATYA JOHANSSON

The list of condiments includes: soy sauce, fish sauce, oyster sauce and tomato paste, a whiff of vinegar, lemon/lime juice, mustard and Worcestershire sauce.
You can have clear soups, miso soup, stock cubes and vegetable soup.

Tomato juice is allowed, about 1/4 of a cup but only a brand that has no added sugar.

Cut down on carbs like white bread, pasta, rice, noodles, potatoes, pumpkin and sweet potatoes, kumara, turnips, corn, peas and beetroot.

Add a bean mix, cannellini beans, red kidney beans, chickpeas, hummus, quinoa, and lentils (a very small quantity) to the diet.

Once the body starts to get resistant to insulin, it can be a difficult process to reverse because of body's resistance to insulin.

Insulin resistance is a common basis for development of glucose intolerance, including diabetes and coronary artery disease, renal disease and blindness.

It is difficult to reverse this condition, but not impossible.

It is possible to reverse insulin resistance and it could take 6 months of hard work, strict diet and exercise, but as said not impossible.

INSULIN RESISTANCE

BREAKFAST RECIPES

1. SOY ZUCCHINI NOODLES RECIPE

INGREDIENTS:

- 2 zucchinis, spiraled
- ½ teaspoon oil

SAUCE:

- ¼ cup soy sauce
- 1 tablespoon of rice vinegar
- 1 tablespoon sesame oil
- ½ teaspoon freshly grated ginger
- toasted sesame seeds

METHOD:

1. For the sauce, combine soy sauce, rice vinegar, sesame oil and grated ginger in a bowl and mix well.
2. Heat ½ teaspoon of oil in a pan and lightly sauté the zucchini noodles for 2 minutes.
3. Remove from heat and add enough of the sauce to coat.
4. Serve hot.

5.

2. PORRIDGE WITH DATES AND HONEY

INGREDIENTS:

- 1 cup Whole Grain Teff
- 1 tablespoon cold Unsalted Butter or Coconut Oil, cut into small pieces
- 1/4 teaspoon ground Cloves
- 3 cups filtered Water
- 1/4 cup Date Pieces or pitted dates (halved crosswise)
- 1/4 teaspoon Sea Salt
- 3 tablespoons to 4 Honey, Maple Syrup or Agave, plus additional for topping
- 1/4 cup Walnuts coarsely chopped (or nut of choice; pecan, almonds, etc.)
- Yogurt, Milk or Cream (optional)

METHOD:

1. Set a heavy, 2-quart saucepan over medium heat. Add the Teff and toast, stirring frequently until the grains emit a mild, toasty aroma and begin to pop, 3 to 6 minutes. (You will notice little white dots of popped grain but may not hear the popping.)
2. Turn off the heat and stand back to avoid sputtering. Add 3 cups of boiling water, the butter, and cloves. Stir well. Turn the heat to medium, cover, and cook at a gentle boil for 10 minutes. Stir from time to time to prevent the grains from sticking to the bottom. Mash any lumps against the side of the pan.
3. Stir in the dates, salt, and honey to taste. Cover and continue cooking until the grains are tender and one

INSULIN RESISTANCE

color throughout (there should be no whitish colored grain).

3. BLUEBERRY AND RASPBERRY MUFFINS

INGREDIENTS:

Dry Ingredients
- 3/4 cup Whole Wheat Flour
- 3/4 cup Oat Bran
- 1/2 cup Brown Sugar
- 1 teaspoon Baking Powder (aluminum free)
- 1/2 teaspoon Baking Soda

Wet Ingredients
- 1 8oz container organic Blueberry Yogurt
- 1 Egg
- 2 tablespoon. Coconut Oil
- 1/2 teaspoon Vanilla
- 1 cup frozen blueberries
- 1 cup frozen raspberries

METHOD:

1. Combine dry ingredients in a bowl.
2. Combine wet ingredients in another bowl.
3. Combine wet with dry and frozen berries.
4. Combine just until all ingredients are well mixed
5. Bake at 400 degrees for 18 minutes.

INSULIN RESISTANCE

4. QUINOA WITH FRESH APPLE

INGREDIENTS:

- 1 cup hot cooked quinoa
- 1/2 unpeeled cubed apple (pink lady, honeycrisp or Fuji)
- 1/4 cup raw almonds
- 1/8 cup raisins
- 1/8-1/4 cup plain almond milk
- 1 tablespoon coconut oil
- Dash of cinnamon
- Drizzle of raw agave syrup

METHOD:

1. Stir all together and eat.

5. OVERNIGHT PROTEIN OATMEAL

INGREDIENTS:

- 3/4 cup unsweetened almond milk (or milk of choice)
- 1/2 cup Plain low fat Greek yogurt (or mashed banana, applesauce or pumpkin)
- 1/2 cup Grated carrots
- 1/4 teaspoon Salt (or to taste)
- 1/2 teaspoon Cinnamon
- 1/2 teaspoon Apple pie spice
- 2 tablespoon Baking stevia (or 1/4 cup sweetener)
- 1 cup Old Fashioned Oats
- 1/4 cup Protein powder (or additional oats)
- Optional: Toppings of choice

METHOD:

1. In a small bowl, mix all of the ingredients together.
2. Divide between 2 small bowls, mugs, or mason jars.
3. Cover and refrigerate overnight (or for at least an hour (or more) so the oats soften and absorb the liquid).
4. Top with chopped nuts, cinnamon, low sugar syrup, or vanilla Greek yogurt if desired.
5. Enjoy cold, or microwave for 30-60 seconds to enjoy warm.

6. CHOCOLATE CHIA OVERNIGHT OATS

INGREDIENTS:

- 2 cups old fashioned oats
- 2 cups milk of your choice (I used soy milk)
- ¼ cup raw cacao powder or cocoa powder
- ¼ cup pure maple syrup
- 3 tablespoons chia seeds

METHOD:

1. In a medium bowl, whisk all ingredients together until well combined.
2. Divide into smaller containers such as mason jars, cover and place in refrigerator overnight.
3. Top with fresh fruit and enjoy!

7. PINEAPPLE MUESLI

INGREDIENTS:

- 3/4 cup pistachios, shells removed and coarsely chopped
- 1/3 cup, unsweetened, flaked coconut
- 1 cup old-fashioned rolled oats
- 1/2 cup chopped dried pineapple
- 1/4 cup wheat bran
- 2 tablespoons chia seeds
- 2 tablespoons Stevia
- 2 tablespoons ground flax seed
- 2 tablespoons oat bran
- 1/8 teaspoon salt
- yogurt or milk, for serving

METHOD:

1. Heat a skillet over medium heat and add the pistachios.
2. Toast for a few minutes, just until slightly golden and fragrant.
3. Pour the pistachios into a large bowl.
4. Add the coconut to the same skillet over medium heat.
5. Stir and shake the pan until the coconut is slightly toasted, about 2 to 3 minutes.
6. Add the coconut to the bowl.

INSULIN RESISTANCE

7.

8. GREEN SMOOTHIE

INGREDIENTS:

- Water as needed
- Almond milk same amount as water
- Coconut water or fresh green juice to taste
- Spinach and kale about a handful of each
- Berries of your choice (about a handful)

ENERGETIC ADD-ONS:
Coconut oil
Ground flax seeds or Chia seeds
Protein powder
Almond butter

METHOD:

1. Add the basic ingredients to you blender and blend until liquefied.
2. How much and how long depends on your blender's power and settings.
3. The best blender is the Blend Tec blender that has a perfect "Smoothie" setting.
4. Next, blend again.
5. Lastly add any more liquid or ice, as desired and blend again, if necessary.

9. SCRAMBLED EGGS WITH SMOKED SALMON

INGREDIENTS:

- 2 eggs
- 1 tablespoon coconut butter
- 1 tablespoon soy milk
- 2 ounces smoked salmon
- Chopped herbs
- Salt and pepper to taste

METHOD:

1. Crack 2 eggs into a small mixing bowl and whisk.
2. Heat a heavy-bottomed nonstick sauté pan over medium-low heat.
3. Add a tablespoon of olive oil or coconut butter.
4. Add a tablespoon of milk to the eggs and season to taste with salt and pepper.
5. Whisk thoroughly to incorporate a bit of air into the mixture.
6. Pour into hot oil or butter and let the eggs cook for up to a minute without stirring to the bottom set.
7. With a rubber spatula, gently push one edge of the egg into the center of the pan, while tilting the pan to allow the still liquid egg to flow in underneath.
8. Repeat with the other edges, until the raw egg is gone.
9. Turn off the heat and continue gently stirring and turning the egg until all the uncooked parts become firm.
10. Don't break up the egg, though. Try to keep the curds as large as possible.
11. Add an ounce or two of smoked salmon and chopped herbs.

INSULIN RESISTANCE

12. Transfer to a plate when the eggs are set but still moist and soft.
13. Eggs are delicate, so they'll continue to cook for a few moments after they're on the plate.

10. AVOCADO SMOOTHIE

INGREDIENTS:

- ½ ripe avocado
- 1 ripe banana
- ½ cup low-fat yogurt
- ½ cup orange juice
- Optional: handful of ice

METHOD:

1. Combine ingredients into blender and mix well.

LUNCH RECIPES

11. CHICKEN PROVENCALE CASSEROLE

INGREDIENTS:

- 300g lean chicken breast, cut into chunks
- 2 tablespoons olive oil
- 2 cloves garlic, minced
- 2 cloves garlic, peeled and whole
- 2 large zucchinis, halved lengthways and cut into chunks
- 6 mushrooms, quartered
- 6 pitted black olives
- 1 small onion chopped
- ½ cup chicken stock
- 1 cup tomato sauce
- 2 spring fresh thyme
- 1 spring tarragon
- 1 spring rosemary
- Handful basil leaves
- Chopped parsley for garnish

METHOD:

1. In an oven proof casserole dish, brown the chicken in olive oil then put aside.
2. In the same casserole dish, lightly sauté the onion, zucchini, mushrooms and minced garlic in olive oil.
3. Add the tomato sauce, chicken stock and herbs.
4. Cover and cook in 160C oven for 30 minutes.
5. Remove cover and cook for another 10 minutes.
6. To serve, sprinkle with chopped parsley.

KATYA JOHANSSON

INSULIN RESISTANCE

12. BAKED SALMON AND MUSSELS IN FOIL

INGREDIENTS:

- 2 x 150g salmon fillet
- 2 teaspoons of olive oil
- Salt and pepper
- 1 zucchini, cut thin lengthwise
- 4 large leaves of bok choy
- 4 black mussels
- 2 cherry tomatoes, halved

METHOD:

1. Preheat oven to 160C.
2. On a large piece of foil, layer the ingredients in the following order: zucchini, bok choy, salmon fillet, salt and pepper, bok choy again, black mussels, cherry tomatoes.
3. Bring the edges of the foil together to form a closed parcel.
4. Bake in the oven for 15 mins.

13. LOW CARB CASSEROLE

INGREDIENTS:

- ½ carrot, cut into thin strips
- ½ zucchini, cut into thin strips
- 2 mushrooms, thinly sliced
- Handful of baby spinach
- 2 shallots cut into thin strips
- 2 strips of dried seaweed cut into thin strips
- ¼ cup cauliflower rice

TO COOK VEGETABLES:
- Sesame oil
- Soy sauce
- Toasted sesame seeds

BULGOGI MARINADE:
- 2 tablespoon soy sauce
- 1 tablespoon sesame oil
- 1 tablespoon Korean chili paste
- 200 g beef, thinly sliced
- 1 egg yolk

METHOD:

1. Cut meat into thin strips and marinade in Bulgogi sauce.
2. Prepare all vegetables.
3. Cook rice and keep warm.
4. Prepare cauliflower rice.
5. Heat a little amount of sesame oil in pan, add each vegetable with a dash of soy sauce and cook on gentle heat for 2-3 minutes.
6. Set aside separately and keep warm.

INSULIN RESISTANCE

7. Heat a little vegetable oil in a pan and stir fry the beef then keep warm.
8. Add a little amount of sesame oil to the same pan and cook rice for 2-3 minutes.
9. Assemble dish: add a little sesame oil on bottom.
10. Top with rice.
11. Add cooked vegetables and meat like spokes of a bicycle wheel.
12. Sprinkle with sesame seeds.
13. Carefully add the egg yolk in the middle.
14. Serve with a side of hot sauce.
15. To serve, mix all together.

14. CHICKEN AND ZUCCHINI

INGREDIENTS:

- 3 medium zucchini, sliced
- 12 ounces chicken breast or tenderloin, chopped
- 1 tablespoon garlic, finely chopped
- 1 tablespoon onion, chopped
- 2 cups sliced mushrooms
- 1/3 cup grated parmesan cheese

METHOD:

1. Spray a skillet or frying pan with cooking spray and turn to medium/high heat.
2. Add onions and garlic, sauté until they begin to turn golden brown.
3. Add the mushrooms and zucchini.
4. Sauté until mushrooms and zucchini start to become tender.
5. Add chicken and continue to sauté on high heat until chicken is completely cooked.
6. Add the parmesan cheese, stirring frequently and coating all the pieces.
7. Remove from heat once cheese has coated all pieces and melted.

INSULIN RESISTANCE

15. EGGPLANT, SQUASH, AND ZUCCHINI CASSEROLE

INGREDIENTS:

- 1.5 Yellow Squash, cut into 1/2" slices
- 1 Medium Zucchini, cut into 1/2" slices
- 5 Medium Eggplants, cut into 1" cubes
- 5 Medium Yellow Onion, chopped
- 2 cloves of Garlic, minced
- 1 10oz can of Rotel (or any other diced tomatoes with chilies)
- 5 cup Canned Diced Tomatoes
- 5 cup grated Parmesan cheese
- 5 cup shredded 2% Mexican Blend cheese
- Butter Flavored Non-Fat Cooking Spray
- Garlic Salt
- Pepper

METHOD:

1. I cooked this in a toaster oven.
2. Preheat oven to 400.
3. Line a baking dish with foil and spray with cooking spray to prevent sticking.
4. Heat large nonstick skillet over medium heat.
5. When skillet is hot, coat with cooking spray.
6. Add onions and garlic.
7. Sautee until soft.
8. Add Rotel, diced tomatoes, eggplant, squash, and zucchini to pan.
9. Sprinkle with garlic salt and pepper to taste.
10. Sautee for 5 minutes.

11. Layer the eggplant/squash mixture and Parmesan, alternating until eggplant mixture is gone.
12. Top with remaining Parmesan or and the Mexican blend cheese.
13. Bake for 20 minutes (or until veggies are cooked to desired doneness).

16. CABBAGE ROLLS

INGREDIENTS:

- 1 medium head cabbage
- 1 1/2 cups uncooked white rice
- 2 tablespoons coconut butter
- 1 Onion, chopped
- Salt and pepper to taste
- 1 (46 fluid ounce) can tomato juice

METHOD:

1. Preheat oven to 325 degrees F (165 degrees C).
2. Grease a 2 quart casserole dish.
3. Steam the whole head of cabbage until it is al dente.
4. Meanwhile, in a saucepan bring 3 cups of water to a boil.
5. Add rice and stir.
6. Reduce heat, cover and simmer for 20 minutes.
7. Melt butter in a small skillet over medium heat.
8. Sauté onion until translucent; stir into cooked rice.
9. Season with salt and pepper to taste.
10. Cut the leaves off of the cabbage and cut the larger leaves in half.
11. Spoon 1 tablespoon of rice into a leaf and roll tightly.
12. Place rolls in prepared casserole dish, stacking in layers.
13. Pour tomato juice over the rolls, using enough just to cover.
14. Cover and bake in preheated oven for 2 hours.

17. STUFFED CABBAGE ROLLS

INGREDIENTS:

- 1 pound ground beef
- 1/2 pound ground pork
- 1 1/2 cups cooked rice
- 1 teaspoon finely chopped garlic
- 1 teaspoon salt, plus more to taste
- 1/4 teaspoon ground black pepper, plus more to taste
- 3 (10.75 ounce) cans condensed tomato soup
- 2 (12 fluid ounce) cans tomato juice, or more to taste
- 1/2 cup ketchup

METHOD:

1. Bring a large pot of lightly salted water to a boil.
2. Place cabbage head into water, cover pot, and cook until cabbage leaves are slightly softened enough to remove from head, 3 minutes.
3. Remove cabbage from pot and let cabbage sit until leaves are cool enough to handle, about 10 minutes.
4. Remove 18 whole leaves from the cabbage head, cutting out any thick tough center ribs. Set whole leaves aside.
5. Chop the remainder of the cabbage head and spread it in the bottom of a casserole dish.
6. Melt butter in a large skillet over medium-high heat.
7. Cook and stir onion in hot butter until tender, 5 to 10 minutes. Cool.
8. Stir onion, beef, pork, rice, garlic, 1 teaspoon salt, and 1/4 teaspoon pepper together in a large bowl.
9. Preheat oven to 350 degrees F (175 degrees C).
10. Place about 1/2 cup beef mixture on a cabbage leaf.

INSULIN RESISTANCE

11. Roll cabbage around beef mixture, tucking in sides to create an envelope around the meat.
12. Repeat with remaining leaves and meat mixture.
13. Place cabbage rolls in a layer atop the chopped cabbage in the casserole dish; season rolls with salt and black pepper.
14. Whisk tomato soup, tomato juice, and ketchup together in a bowl.
15. Pour tomato soup mixture over cabbage rolls and cover dish wish aluminum foil.
16. Bake in the preheated oven until cabbage is tender and meat is cooked through, about 1 hour.

18. STUFFED MUSHROOMS

INGREDIENTS:

- 48 fresh whole baby portabella or white mushrooms (1 1/2 to 2 inches in diameter)
- 1 package (8 oz.) cream cheese, softened
- 1 box (9 oz.) frozen chopped spinach, thawed, squeezed to drain
- 1 cup freshly grated Parmesan cheese
- 1/2 teaspoon salt
- 1/4 teaspoon freshly ground black pepper
- 1/8 teaspoon ground red pepper (cayenne)
- 1/2 cup panko crispy bread crumbs
- 2 tablespoons butter melted

METHOD:

1. Heat oven to 350°F.
2. Remove stems from mushroom caps; reserve caps.
3. Discard stems.
4. In large bowl, mix cream cheese, spinach, 1/2 cup of the Parmesan cheese, the salt and both peppers until well blended.
5. Spoon into mushroom caps, mounding slightly.
6. Place mushrooms in ungreased 17x12-inch half-sheet pan.
7. In small bowl, mix remaining 1/2 cup Parmesan cheese, the bread crumbs and butter.
8. Sprinkle bread crumb mixture over filled mushroom caps, pressing lightly.
9. Bake 20 to 22 minutes or until thoroughly heated.
10. Serve immediately.

19. SLOW-COOKER POT ROAST

INGREDIENTS:

- 8 small red potatoes cut in half
- 3-pound beef boneless arm roast, trimmed of fat
- 2 tablespoons all-purpose flour
- 1 pound baby-cut carrots
- 1 jar (16 ounces) Old El Paso Thick 'n Chunky salsa

METHOD:

1. Place potatoes in 3 1/2- to 4-quart slow cooker.
2. Coat beef with flour; place on potatoes.
3. Arrange carrots around beef.
4. Pour salsa over all.
5. Cover and cook on low heat setting 8 to 10 hours.
6. Remove beef from cooker; place on cutting board.
7. Pull beef into serving pieces, using 2 forks.
8. To serve, spoon sauce over beef and vegetables.

20. ZUCCHINI PARMESAN

INGREDIENTS:

- 1 cup sliced zucchini
- 1 tablespoon shredded Parmesan cheese
- 10 squirts butter spray

METHOD:

1. Line a cookie sheet with aluminum foil, then coat with some cooking spray.
2. Place the zucchini slices out on the pan, then spritz with them with the butter spray.
3. Sprinkle on the parmesan cheese and then pop it in the oven.
4. Broil for a few minutes - until the cheese starts to brown.
5. Enjoy it while it's warm!

Dinner Recipes

21. ITALIAN STYLE COD

INGREDIENTS:

- 400g cod fillets
- 2 tablespoon grated Pecorino Romano cheese
- 2 tablespoon grated Parmesan cheese
- 2 cloves of garlic, crushed
- 50g butter, melted
- 1 tablespoon fresh parsley, finely chopped
- Salt and pepper to taste

METHOD:

1. Preheat the oven to Gas Mark 6 or 200°C.
2. Lightly grease an ovenproof dish.
3. Mix the cheeses, garlic and seasoning in a bowl.
4. Place the fillets in the ovenproof dish and cover with the cheese mixture and parsley.
5. Season to taste.
6. Bake for 15 minutes and serve immediately.

22. LAMB KEBABS

INGREDIENTS:

KEBAB MIX
- 400g minced lamb
- 2 teaspoon. garlic, peeled and finely chopped
- 2 teaspoon. ginger, peeled and finely chopped
- 1 large onion, peeled and finely chopped
- 2 teaspoon ground coriander
- 2 teaspoon ground cumin
- ¼ teaspoon ground black pepper
- 1 tablespoon fresh coriander, finely chopped
- 4 metal skewers

GREEN SALSA MIX
- 3 spring onions, chopped
- 1 tablespoon olive oil
- 4 tomatoes, chopped roughly
- 1 tablespoon pitted olives of your choice
- 1 bunch of coriander, chopped
- 1 bunch of parsley, chopped
- Juice and grated rind of a lemon

METHOD:
1. Mix the mince, onion, ginger, garlic, coriander, cumin, pepper and salt in a mixing bowl.
2. Form 16 balls out of the mince mixture.

INSULIN RESISTANCE

3. Put each ball around the tip of a metal skewer and flatten slightly.
4. Place the meatballs on a baking sheet and cover and then refrigerate them for an hour.
5. Pop all the salsa ingredients a bowl and mix together.
6. Cook the skewered lamb kebabs under a preheated grill, turning every now and again, until the lamb is cooked through.
7. This will take 15 minutes.
8. Serve hot with the salsa.

23. SALMON AND BROCCOLI

INGREDIENTS:

- 4 salmon fillets weighing 460g
- 1 head of broccoli
- 1 red chili, finely chopped
- 400ml half fat single cream
- 1 tablespoon. tomato purée
- 100g red pesto
- Freshly ground pepper to taste

METHOD:

1. Preheat the oven to Gas Mark 5 or 190°C.
2. Mix the cream, tomato puree and red pesto together.
3. Then add in the chopped red chili.
4. Place the broccoli and the salmon in the red pesto sauce in 4 individual pot pie dishes, ensuring the fish is fully coated, and bake in the preheated oven for 20 minutes.
5. Remove from the oven and allow cooling for 5 minutes or so and serve.

INSULIN RESISTANCE

24. STUFFED TURKEY BREAST

INGREDIENTS:

- 2 tablespoon olive oil
- 2 medium onions
- 6 garlic cloves, finely chopped
- Salt and pepper to season
- 6 x 200g turkey breasts (opt for a thicker breast in order to fillet it easier)
- 180g cheddar cheese, grated
- 100g gruyere cheese, grated
- 12 slices Parma ham
- Steamed broccoli and cauliflower
- Juice of a lemon

METHOD:

1. Pour a tablespoon of olive oil into a saucepan and place over a medium heat until the oil warms up.
2. Sauté the onions for around 4 minutes, add the garlic and cook for another 2 minutes.
3. Season the mixture with salt and pepper, then set it aside to cool down.
4. Partly fillet the turkey breast.
5. You should open up the turkey enough to make a small pocket and then stuff the cheddar and gruyere inside that pocket.
6. Season the turkey breasts with salt and pepper, and wrap two slices of Parma ham around each breast.
7. Drizzle the turkey breasts with the rest of the olive oil and bake at 180°c or Gas Mark 4 for 25 minutes, ensuring that the ham is crispy and the chicken is fully cooked.

8. To test if the turkey is cooked, stick a skewer in it: when it comes out, the juice should be clear and not be at all pink.
9. Serve along with steamed broccoli and cauliflower, dressed with some lemon juice.

25. EGGPLANT RATATOUILLE

INGREDIENTS:

- 2 tablespoons extra virgin olive oil
- 2 onions chopped
- 4 cloves garlic minced
- 2 eggplants peeled in strips and cut into 3/4 inch cubes
- 4 zucchini cut into 1 inch cubes
- Salt and pepper to taste
- 3 bell peppers red or yellow (ribs and seeds removed, cut into 3/4 inch cubes)
- 1 can diced tomatoes
- 1 teaspoon dried thyme
- 1/2 cup basil chopped

METHOD:

1. In a large pot with a snug-fitting lid), heat oil over medium heat.
2. Cook onions and stir occasionally until soft, about 5 minutes.
3. Add garlic; cook until aromatic, about 1 minute.
4. Stir in eggplant and zucchini; season with salt and pepper to taste.
5. Add 3/4 cup water; cover, and simmer until vegetables begin to soften, stirring once, about 5 minutes.
6. Add bell peppers, stir; simmer and cover until softened, 5 minutes.
7. Stir in tomatoes and thyme; bring to a boil.
8. Reduce heat to medium-low.
9. Partially cover; simmer, until vegetables are tender (stirring often), about 15 to 20 minutes.
10. Remove from heat.

KATYA JOHANSSON

26. QUICK MADE PORK

INGREDIENTS:

- tablespoon water
- 1 tablespoon Worcestershire sauce for chicken
- 1 teaspoon lemon juice
- 1 teaspoon Dijon-style mustard
- 4 3 - ounces boneless pork top loin chops, cut 3/4 to 1 inch thick
- 1/2-1 teaspoon lemon-pepper seasoning
- 1 tablespoon butter or margarine
- 1 tablespoon snipped fresh chives, parsley, or oregano

METHOD:

1. For sauce, in a small bowl stir together the water, Worcestershire sauce, lemon juice, and mustard;
2. Set aside.
3. Trim fat from chops.
4. Sprinkle both sides of each chop with lemon-pepper seasoning.
5. In a 10-inch skillet melt butter over medium heat.
6. Add chops and cook for 8 to 12 minutes or until pork juices run clear (160 degrees F), turning once halfway through cooking time.
7. Remove from heat.
8. Transfer chops to a serving platter; cover with foil and keep warm.
9. Pour sauce into skillet; stir to scrape up any crusty browned bits from bottom of skillet.
10. Pour sauce over chops.
11. Sprinkle with chives.

27. CHICKEN AND APPLE BURGERS

INGREDIENTS:

Burgers
- 1 lb. (500 g) ground chicken
- 1 large red onion, finely chopped
- 1/4 cup (50 mL) plain dry bread crumbs
- 2 large green apples, such as Granny Smith (for a tart taste) or Golden Delicious (for a sweet taste), peeled and coarsely grated
- 1 tablespoon (15 mL) chopped fresh sage leaves
- 1 tablespoon (15 mL) fresh thyme leaves
- 1/4 teaspoon (1 mL) salt
- 1/4 teaspoon (1 mL) freshly ground black pepper

To Serve
- 1/4 cup (50 mL) Dijon mustard
- 1 tablespoon (15 mL) honey
- 4 whole-wheat hamburger buns, split
- 6 tablespoon (90 mL) watercress sprigs

METHOD:

1. In a large bowl, place the chicken, onion, bread crumbs, apples, sage, thyme, salt and pepper. Using your hands, mix the ingredients together until the ingredients are distributed evenly throughout. Wet your hands, then divide the mixture into 4 equal portions and shape each into a burger about 4 in. (10 cm) in diameter and 1 1/2 in. (4 cm) thick. Chill the burgers for 1 hour to firm up the meat and make it easier to hold together while it cooks.

2. Preheat the grill or broiler to high. Place burgers on a rack about 6 in. (15 cm) from the source of heat. Grill or broil the burgers, turning them once, until they are golden brown on both sides and until they are still juicy but cooked through completely.
3. While the burgers cook, mix the mustard and honey in a small cup. On a flat surface, open the 4 buns with the soft cut sides up. Spread the honey mustard on cut sides of both the tops and bottoms of the buns. Pile one fourth of the watercress on the bottom of each bun.
4. When the burgers are ready, transfer a burger to the bottom of each bun, placing it on top of the watercress. Cover with the top of the bun and serve immediately

28. SALMON AND ASPARAGUS

INGREDIENTS:

- 4 skinless salmon fillets (about 4 oz/125 g each)
- 2 leeks, thinly sliced
- 8 oz. (250 g) asparagus spears
- 1 cup (250 mL) sugar snap peas
- 4 tablespoon (60 mL) dry white wine
- 1 cup (250 mL) reduced-sodium vegetable broth
- Salt and pepper

METHOD:

1. Run your fingertips over each salmon fillet to check for stray bones, pulling out any that remain.
2. Arrange the leeks in a single layer in the bottom of a large Dutch oven coated with cooking spray.
3. Lay the pieces of salmon on top.
4. Surround the fish with the asparagus and peas. Add the wine and broth, and season lightly with salt and pepper.
5. Place the Dutch oven over medium-high heat and bring broth to a boil, then cover with a tight-fitting lid and reduce the heat to low.
6. Cook the fish and vegetables until the salmon is pale pink all the way through and the vegetables are tender, about 12 to 14 minutes.
7. Sprinkle the chives over the salmon and serve.

29. HIGH FIBER BREAD

INGREDIENTS:

- Works in a bread machine, regular cycle.
- 1 slice = 1 Carb
- One loaf makes about 12 slices.
- 2 cups rye flour
- 2 tablespoon wheat gluten
- 1/2 cup oat bran
- 1/4 cup rolled oats
- 1/4 cup flax meal, more bran, or 9-grain cereal
- 1 tablespoon honey
- 1 tablespoon olive oil
- 1 teaspoon salt
- 1 teaspoon bread yeast
- 1 teaspoon caraway or nigella seeds for added flavor
- 1 and 1/4 cup lukewarm water

METHOD:

1. By adding the gluten, you can get away with using a much higher percentage of whole grain and fiber while still getting dough that rises in a bread machine.
2. By following a basic ratio of 2 cups whole flour (wheat, rye, oat, etc.) to 1 cup coarser ingredients (wheat, oat, or rice bran, 9 grain cereal, rolled oats, seeds, etc.) along with that extra gluten, the bread usually turns out firm and dense, but not leaden or overly dry.
3. You might need to adjust the amount of water by a tablespoon or two depending on your choice of grains.
4. The honey helps the yeast rise, so adding a bit more makes more porous bread.

5. The oil helps prevent the bread from drying out after baking, so the loaf retains a fresh texture for several days after baking.
6. If baking this by hand, knead for about 10 minutes, let rise for two hours, gently punch down, let rise again for an hour, and bake for about an hour at 350 F.

INSULIN RESISTANCE

30. TILAPIA, MUSHROOM DUXELLES

INGREDIENTS:

DUXELLES:
- 1/2 lb. fresh mushrooms, finely chopped
- 1 onion, finely chopped
- 1 tablespoon olive oil
- 1/2 teaspoon salt
- 1/2 cup chicken stock
- black pepper to taste

TILAPIA:
- 1 tilapia fillet per person
- Splash of dry vermouth
- 1 clove of garlic
- 1 teaspoon olive oil
- Pinch of salt, pepper, nutmeg

METHOD:

1. Heat a large skillet on medium, spread oil onto it, then add onions and mushrooms.
2. Stir occasionally while reducing liquid out of the blend, on medium-low heat, for 30-60 minutes.
3. You don't need to attend it constantly, just make sure it doesn't brown too much or burn.
4. As the blend becomes dry, add stock and salt to taste (if stock is unsalted.)
5. Grind in some fresh pepper.
6. Continue to reduce until flavors are very concentrated, and texture becomes somewhat homogenized.

7. Set aside
8. Vegetables: before starting the fish, chop up some green winter vegetables and put them in a covered ceramic dish, for the microwave.
9. Splash with dry vermouth or white wine (or water-lemon juice mix) and microwave for a few minutes, just before serving.
10. For this dinner I used bok choy, Asparagus and Romanesco.
11. Many choices could work as accompaniment, such as spinach, broccoli, chard, etc.
12. Before serving the vegetables, sprinkle them with a good balsamic vinegar, salt and pepper.
13. Heat a large heavy skillet, with a lid nearby.
14. Finely mince a clove of garlic. Sprinkle salt and pepper over thawed tilapia fillets.
15. Spread olive oil on skillet, and place tilapia on medium-high heat for a minute or two on one side.
16. Flip the fish fillets carefully onto the other side, so as not to break them apart.
17. Toss in the garlic and wait a moment to let it sear.
18. While searing the garlic, sprinkle a tiny pinch of nutmeg or mace onto the upper side of each fillet.
19. Now add a splash of dry vermouth (or a un-oaked white wine) to deglaze the pan and prevent the garlic from burning.
20. Once the alcohol has evaporated out of the liquid (a minute or two) put the lid on the pan and reduce heat, to steam a moment while plating the rest of the meal.
21. Plate the tilapia atop a couple tablespoons of Duxelles, alongside a large pile of vegetables, and with a sprinkling of parsley and green onions.

Desserts

31. MOLTEN CHOCOLATE CAKES

INGREDIENTS:

- 4 tablespoon butter, plus extra for buttering ramekins
- 6 squares Lindt 85% cacao chocolate
- 1 large egg
- 1 egg yolk
- 1 tablespoon granulated erythritol
- 1 teaspoon flour

METHOD:

1. Preheat oven to 450F and butter two 4oz ramekins well.
2. Dust ramekins with cocoa powder and set aside.
3. Melt butter and chocolate together in a small bowl set over a pan of simmering water.
4. Stir until smooth.
5. In a medium bowl, beat egg, egg yolk and erythritol together until lightened in color and thickened.
6. Add chocolate mixture and mix until combined.
7. Stir in flour.
8. Divide between ramekins.
9. At this point, you could cover and chill for later, just bring back to room temperature before baking.
10. Bake 6-7 minutes.
11. Sides will be set but center will still be soft.
12. Invert onto a plate and let sit for 10 seconds or so, then lift one side of ramekin.
13. Cake will fall out onto plate.

14. Serve immediately.

INSULIN RESISTANCE

32. NO SUGAR OAT DROPS

INGREDIENTS:

- 1 1/2 cups regular rolled oats (use whatever type of oats you like)
- 1 cup coconut flakes
- 1/2 teaspoon salt
- 1 teaspoon cinnamon
- 1/2 teaspoon allspice
- 1/4 cup of almond meal (or nutmeal of your choice)
- 1/2 cup mixed nuts, finely chopped
- 1 cup dried fruit (of your choice or chocolate chips or berries)
- 3 ripe bananas, mashed (or substitute applesauce, or 2 eggs)
- 1/4 cup canola oil (or oil of your choice)
- 1 teaspoon vanilla extract

METHOD:

1. Preheat oven to 175C.
2. Line baking sheet with parchment paper.
3. In a large bowl, combine rolled oats, almond meal, mixed nuts and coconut flakes. Stir in allspice and cinnamon.
4. Add dried fruit and stir until well and evenly mixed.
5. Make sure the dried fruit do not stick together in big batches.
6. In another bowl, combine canola oil, mashed banana and vanilla extract.
7. Pour wet ingredients over dry ingredients and stir until well combined.

8. Take a large cookie cutter and press gently spoonfuls of the batter into it.
9. Remove cookie cutter.
10. Or simply form balls with your hands and flatten slightly.
11. Bake for about 20 minutes or until edges are golden brown.

33. ALMOND BUTTER CHOCOLATE CHIP COOKIES

INGREDIENTS:

- 2 ripe bananas, mashed
- 1-cup natural almond butter
- 2 tablespoons real maple syrup
- 2 cups oats
- ½ teaspoon sea salt
- ½ cup dark chocolate chips

METHOD:

1. Preheat oven to 350 F
2. In a small glass bowl, mash bananas, and stir in almond butter.
3. Microwave for 30 seconds to melt the mixture, and bring out the banana flavor.
4. Stir in maple syrup.
5. In a large bowl, combine oats and sea salt.
6. Add banana mixture to oats, and stir to combine.
7. Fold in chocolate chips.
8. Line a cookie sheet with parchment paper, and spoon out cookie dough (about 2 tbsp. per cookie).
9. Bake for 10 – 15 minutes.
10. Let cool on the cookie sheet.
11. Store in the freezer.

34. CHOCOLATE PEANUT BUTTER FUDGE

INGREDIENTS:

- ¾ cup coconut oil, melted
- 2/3-cup honey
- ¾ cup cocoa powder
- ½ cup all-natural peanut butter
- 1 tablespoon vanilla extract
- ½ teaspoon sea salt

OPTIONAL ADDITIONS:
- Raw cacao nibs
- Pumpkin seeds
- Unsweetened shredded coconut
- Hemp seeds
- Walnuts
- Slivered almonds

METHOD:

1. Melt the coconut oil in a large Pyrex measuring cup.
2. Once melted, whisk in honey, cocoa powder, peanut butter, vanilla and sea salt.
3. Pour the mixture into a parchment lined loaf pan and chill in the fridge for 1-2 hours or until completely set.
4. Cut into squares, and store in the fridge or freezer.

35. CARAMEL MACCHIATO CHEESECAKES

INGREDIENTS:

FOR THE CHEESECAKES:
- 8 oz. cream cheese, softened
- 2 tablespoon unsalted butter
- 3 eggs
- 3 tablespoon Cold Brew Coffee Concentrate (or espresso)
- 1 tablespoon sugar free caramel flavored syrup see example
- ⅓ Cup granulated sugar substitute (Swerve, Splenda, Ideal, etc.)

FOR THE FROSTING:
- 3 tablespoon unsalted butter, softened
- 3 tablespoon sugar free caramel flavored syrup see example
- 2 tablespoon granulated sugar substitute (Swerve, Splenda, Ideal, etc)
- 8oz Mascarpone cheese, softened

METHOD:

1. For the cheesecakes: combine all of the cheesecake ingredients in a magic bullet or blender.
2. Blend until smooth.
3. Pour into 9 greased silicone cupcake molds, or in a cupcake pan lined with paper liners.
4. Bake at 350 degrees (F) for 15 minutes or until firm when shaken slightly.
5. Remove and chill for one hour in the freezer or at least 3 hours (preferably overnight) in the refrigerator.

6. For the frosting: cream the butter, sugar free caramel syrup, and sweetener together until fluffy.
7. At a low speed (or it will break), blend in the mascarpone until smooth.
8. Test and adjust for desired sweetness.
9. If your frosting breaks, add a few tablespoons of regular cream cheese to stabilize it.
10. Pipe or spoon onto your chilled cheesecakes before serving.

36. CHEESE MOUSSE AND BERRIES

INGREDIENTS:

- 8 ounces mascarpone cheese
- 1 cup whipping cream
- 3/4 teaspoon vanilla stevia drops
- Berries (1 pint blueberries and 1 pint strawberries)

METHOD:

1. Whip together mascarpone, cream, and sweetener in large mixing bowl with electric mixer until stiff peaks form.
2. Pipe into individual cups and layer with berries

37. LEMON GELATIN DESSERT

INGREDIENTS:

- 3 1/3 cups = 800 ml filtered water
- 3 bags Lemon Zinger herbal tea
- 1/2 cup = 120 ml powdered erythritol
- 30 drops Lemon Twist stevia
- 3 tablespoons freshly squeezed juice from organic lemon
- 1 1/2 tablespoons unflavored grass-fed gelatin powder

METHOD:

1. Heat 3 cups (710 ml) of the water until boiling.
2. Add the teabags and the sweeteners. Let cool to room temperature and remove the tea bags, gently squeezing to save all the liquid.
3. Take the rest (1/3 cup ≈ 80 ml) of the water and pour it into a microwave safe cup.
4. Add the lemon juice. Sprinkle the gelatin powder on top.
5. Set for 10 minutes.
6. Heat the gelatin mixture in a microwave until steaming hot but not boiling. Mix to ensure that the entire gelatin is dissolved.
7. Pour the hot gelatin mixture into the tea mixture, constantly stirring.
8. Set aside.
9. Spray or brush gelatin molds with light olive oil. You can also use a silicone tube pan.
10. After the gelatin is dissolved in the tea mixture, pour the mixture into the gelatin molds or the silicone tube pan.
11. Refrigerate for 6 hours, or until set.
12. Before serving, rinse the bottom of the molds under hot, running water.
13. Notice that no dessert should get in touch with the hot water.

14. Carefully remove the gelatin from the molds: place a serving plate upside down on top of a mold.
15. Hold both the mold and the serving plate tightly together and quickly turn over the whole thing.
16. Remove extremely carefully the mold, ensuring that the gelatin comes out nicely and completely.
17. Repeat with the rest of the molds.
18. Decorate if you wish, and serve immediately.
19. Store the leftovers in the fridge.

38. STRAWBERRY COCONUT POPSICLES

INGREDIENTS:

- 1.25 cups Strawberries, fresh or frozen
- 1 tablespoon Liquid Stevia, or Local Honey
- 1 teaspoon Vanilla Extract
- ¾ cup Coconut Milk, from a can

METHOD:

1. Optional: Defrost frozen berries the night before.
2. Place the strawberries, vanilla extract, coconut milk and stevia or honey in a blender.
3. Blend ingredients until combined.
4. Pour into Popsicle molds (6X).
5. Freeze for at least 6 hours

39. CHOCOLATE BLACK FOREST TRIFLE

INGREDIENTS:

- 1 8 oz. package no-sugar-added low-fat chocolate cake mix
- 1 large sugar-free instant chocolate pudding mix
- 2 cups fat-free milk
- 1-pound fresh cherries (pitted), or frozen cherries, thaw and drain before preparing recipe.
- 2 cups thawed fat free dessert topping (cool Whip)
- Optional topping: unsweetened cocoa powder

METHOD:

1. Prepare cake mix according to directions on the package using the 8-inch square or round cake pan method.
2. Cool prepared cake for 10 minutes
3. Remove cake from pan and cut into ten 1-inch pieces.
4. Prepare the pudding while the cake bakes according to package directions but use 2 cups fat-free milk.
5. Cover prepared pudding and chill for 30 minutes.
6. A trifle is a layer, so you will need to layer the cake, cherries, and frozen topping into a 3-quart trifle bowl.
7. You can make less thick layers, or more thin layers.
8. Thin typically works best.
9. Continue to layer until you run out of cake and the final layer should be the frozen topping.
10. Sprinkle chocolate shavings or cocoa powder if desired.

40. LOW-SUGAR BROWNIES

INGREDIENTS:

- 3 tablespoon. Nutiva Organic Coconut Flour, sifted
- ¼ cup natural cocoa powder
- ¼ teaspoon sea salt 1 cup creamy almond butter, sunflower seed butter or macadamia nut butter
- 1 teaspoon organic vanilla extract
- 1 tsp. grass-fed gelatin
- 2 tablespoons Enjoy Life Dark Chocolate Morsels, melted
- 2 tablespoons Navitas Naturals Organic Palm Sugar (Coconut Sugar)
- 4 tablespoon Wholesome Sweeteners Organic Zero (Erythritol)
- ½ teaspoon baking soda
- 10 tablespoon filtered water
- 1 teaspoon liquid stevia (to taste)
- ½ teaspoon baking powder -

METHOD:

1. Preheat oven to 325 F.
2. Line the bottom of an 8-by-8 pan with unbleached parchment paper.
3. In a medium bowl, combine the coconut flour, coconut sugar, erythritol, cocoa powder, baking powder, baking soda and salt.
4. In a small bowl, add the water and sprinkle over the gelatin.
5. Let stand 5 minutes.
6. Add almond butter (or "nut" butter of choice), vanilla, stevia and melted chocolate.
7. Mix well using a hand-held mixer.
8. Pour in the dry ingredients and mix well to combine.

9. Spread brownie batter into prepared pan.
10. Transfer to oven and bake 30-35 minutes or until edges pull away and center is set.
11. If you like your brownies fudgy and moist inside, remove when center is still smoothly, at about 30 minutes.
12. Place on a wire rack to cool completely, then slice into squares.

CONCLUSION

I really hope you liked this book and all the recipes in it.

I would like to take this opportunity and thank you for purchasing my eBook.

It means a lot to me and I hope you'll find more books you like from my list above.

Please take a few minutes to leave a kind review on amazon, as it can help my brand grow and allow me to get more books out there each month.

Sincerely yours,

Katya.